The Essential
DEMENTIA
CARE
Handbook

Additional titles in the **Winslow Editions** series:

Accent Method: A Rational Voice Therapy in Theory & Practice,
Kirsten Thyme-Frøkjær & Børge Frøkjær-Jensen

Beyond Aphasia: Therapies for Living with Communication Disability,
Carole Pound, Susie Parr, Jayne Lindsay & Celia Woolf

Challenging Behaviour in Dementia: A person-centred approach, Graham Stokes

Counselling with Reality Therapy, Robert E Wubbolding & John Brickell

Elder Abuse: Therapeutic Perspectives in Practice, Andrew Papadopoulos &
Jenny la Fontaine

Family Therapy with Older Adults & their Families, Alison Marriott

Human Communication: A Linguistic Introduction, Graham Williamson

Manual of AAC Assessment, Arlene McCurtin & Geraldine Murray

Person-Centred Approaches to Dementia Care, Ian Morton

The Essential
DEMENTIA
CARE
Handbook

Graham
Stokes

Fiona
Goudie

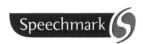

Speechmark Publishing Ltd
Telford Road, Bicester, Oxon OX26 4LQ, UK

Published by
Speechmark Publishing Ltd, Telford Road, Bicester, Oxon OX26 4LQ, UK
www.speechmark.net

© Graham Stokes & Fiona Goudie, 2002

First published 2002

002-4254/Printed in the United Kingdom/1010

British Library Cataloguing in Publication Data
The essential dementia care handbook. – (Winslow editions)
   1. Dementia   2. Dementia – Patients – Care
   I. Stokes, Graham, 1952–   II. Goudie, Fiona
   362.1'9'683

ISBN 0 86388 244 7

Contents

Tables

Figures

Contributors

Pam Enderby

Professor Pam Enderby qualified as a speech and language therapist in 1970. She has since combined clinical work with research. She was appointed Professor of Community Rehabilitation, Sheffield University, in 1996 and combined this post with that of Head of the Department of Human Communication Sciences until September 2000. She has led research programmes into various aspects of therapy, particularly related to models of delivery, effectiveness and outcomes, and has published broadly. She is currently Dean of the Faculty of Medicine at the University of Sheffield.

Fiona Goudie

Fiona Goudie is a consultant clinical psychologist. She has been Head of Older Adult Clinical Psychology Services with Psychological Health Sheffield since 1992. Her research and publications focus on depression and psychological therapies in dementia care. She co-edited *Working with Dementia* (Speechmark, 1990) with Graham Stokes.

Una Holden

Una Holden is a consultant clinical psychologist and Fellow of the British Psychological Society. After qualifying she worked in the USA, returning to develop neurology services for older adults in Leeds. She was instrumental in introducing reality orientation to the UK and, with Bob

Woods, published the first edition of *Reality Orientation* in 1982. She has written numerous articles and several books. Following a time as Senior Lecturer at Plymouth University, she became Head of Clincal Psychology Services for Elderly People in Carlisle and delivered training courses and lectured in the UK, the USA, Canada, Singapore and mainland Europe. Una currently works as a freelance consultant from her home in Spain.

Carolien Lamers

Carolien Lamers is a social gerontologist and clinical psychologist who has been working in Britain for 12 years. She has published on issues of carers' support and interventions. One of her main interests is the diagnostic work undertaken in a memory clinic, and communication with clients regarding their experience of the condition, either individually or in groups.

Ian Morton

Ian Morton is a nurse who has worked with people with dementia for more than 15 years, currently as the manager of a day centre in Eastwood, Nottinghamshire. He has written extensively on approaches to interacting with people with dementia, which draw in the different psychotherapeutic traditions, and in 1999 his book *Person-Centred Approaches to Dementia Care* was published by Speechmark.

Tessa Perrin

Tessa Perrin is an occupational therapist with 15 years' experience of the dementia care field in both health and social service settings. She is currently Director of Training for the National Association for Providers of Activities for Older People. She is author and co-author of numerous articles and books on therapeutic activity and dementia care.

Marie Claire Shankland

Marie Claire Shankland is a consultant clinical psychologist in Sheffield. Her professional interests are working with carers of people with dementia and psychotherapy with older adults.

Graham Stokes

Graham Stokes is Consultant Clinical Psychologist at South Staffordshire Healthcare NHS Trust and Consultant Director of Mental Health at BUPA Care Homes. His interests are in neuropsychology and the understanding and resolution of challenging behaviour in dementia. He has been instrumental in the development of person-centred approaches to care. He has written extensively on the psychology of late life, dementia and person-centred care, including *On Being Old: The Psychology of Later Life* (Routledge Falmer, 1992) and *Challenging Behaviour in Dementia* (Speechmark, 2000) and, with Fiona Goudie, he co-edited *Working with Dementia* (Speechmark, 1990).

John Wattis

Professor John Wattis was appointed Visiting Professor of Psychiatry in Older Adults at Huddersfield University in 2000. Before this he pioneered old-age psychiatry services as a consultant and senior lecturer in Leeds. His published research has been in the development of old-age psychiatry, alcohol abuse and mental illness in geriatric medicine. He has written books and numerous chapters on these topics.

Preface

DEMENTIA REMAINS A TERRIBLE AFFLICTION with no prospect of cure. Yet in so many ways this book resonates optimism and hope for the future. Not because genetics or medicine are about to offer us a way out of a human tragedy that affects so many. Instead, our confidence is founded on the awareness that so much that was once seen as symptoms of disease, and hence impossible to redress or overcome, is better interpreted as the efforts of a person trying to live their life in the midst of intellectual turmoil. We appreciate that the person and their experience matters. A subjective world of belief, knowledge and feeling that was historically not simply ignored by many practitioners and carers, its existence was not even acknowledged.

Was dementia not a terrible illness that destroys the person, leaving behind a body, shell or shadow (you could take your pick)? Nowadays, we know the person has not departed, and so our understanding focuses less on the mechanics of the brain and the effects of pathology on cognition and function, and more on strengths, needs and emotions.

This feels quite different from the time, 12 years ago, when we edited the book *Working with Dementia* (Stokes & Goudie, 1990). Initially this volume was to be a revised edition of that original work – a book that had called for all to be concerned with more than diseased brains. We realised, however, that the ideas being expressed and the practices now being reported had progressed far from the green shoots of person-centred care described in the original book (see for example, p170). A new book was in preparation.

In *The Essential Dementia Care Handbook* we have set ourselves the task of distancing ourselves from the limitations placed on our understanding by neurology and organic psychiatry – what Kitwood (1989) referred to as the 'standard paradigm'. This book is about *people* with dementia; written for practitioners who wish to learn about the ways of those who look at the world through 'worried eyes' (Cheston & Bender, 1999).

The past decade has seen a dramatic growth in the literature on person-centred approaches to dementia care (eg, Kitwood & Bredin, 1992; Kitwood, 1997; Cheston & Bender, 1999; Morton, 1999; Stokes, 2000; Benson, 2000). We hope this book consolidates these conceptual shifts and progresses further the insights that are transforming our contemporary understanding of dementia. The medical model is not rejected, but we advance from pathology to person and enter the realm of interpersonal relationships to ask the question 'How well do I truly know what this person needs and how able am I to meet those needs?' We consider the interactions between the person with dementia and their family and caregivers, and question the role these play in the experience of dementia.

We hope by the end of the book the reader will have been helped to appreciate the contributions of humanistic and social psychology to our understanding of dementia, and the value of psychological therapy to addressing the emotional trauma so often present. To assist us in these objectives, whenever possible we have employed case profiles to bring life to the principles and procedures we advocate.

While much of the content of *The Essential Dementia Care Handbook* is refreshingly new, we have kept a similar structure to *Working with Dementia*. In Part One, 'Setting The Scene', Fiona Goudie starts with her reflections on a decade of vibrant clinical and research activity. Una Holden and Graham Stokes then describe the neuropathology of dementia, demonstrating that while the 'public face' of dementia is Alzheimer's disease there is much more to consider. In Chapter 3, Fiona Goudie stays within the biomedical realm and considers illnesses common in later life that mimic dementia and can result in a problem of differential diagnosis.

Part Two is concerned with 'Discovery', and explores the issues of assessment and understanding that take us beyond the medical model.

Fiona Goudie describes the tools employed to assess a person's strengths and difficulties, revealing how assessment enables us to describe accurately intellectual and self-care abilities, and how descriptions can inform care plans and assist the process of diagnosis. The contribution of assessment to accurate diagnosis is described by Carolien Lamers in her chapter on 'Memory Clinics' – multi-professional diagnostic resources that have become increasingly available throughout the UK during the 1990s and provide for many people their first contact with specialists in cognitive impairment and dementia. The remaining chapters in 'Discovery' set a different tone by concentrating on the person and the conviction that so much of what we observe in dementia is the function of human relationships. Graham Stokes considers what is meant by a person-centred approach to dementia and writes of the person's possible subjective experience. In Chapter 6, a person-centred model of understanding is presented – a framework that develops a central tenant of the book. We work with people who have dementia; people with whom we share far more in common than that which separates us. The person is placed in the context of their environment, not so much the buildings within which they live, but more importantly the context of social relations. In the final chapter in this section, Graham Stokes introduces the methodology of functional analysis. Order is placed on the complex tapestry of explanation, helping us to understand why a person behaves the way they do, when they do and what meaning their behaviour has for them.

In the third section – 'Relearning and Rehabilitation' – we attempt to demonstrate the value of the 're' words – what Kitwood (1989) termed 'rementia'. We hope this section helps people to re-frame dementia by disputing the inevitable remorselessness of decline and degeneration. Advancing and eventually total dependency is inevitable, but realistic goals and actions may slow down deterioration demonstrably and at times restore skills that were thought to be lost. Una Holden and Graham Stokes examine the potential of neuropsychological rehabilitation, having first described specific relationships between brain and behaviour. In Chapter 10, Pam Enderby examines the contribution speech therapy can make to assisting communication in dementia. Graham Stokes then explores the challenge of toileting difficulties, illustrating the value of promoting the goal of assisted independence. The final chapter in this section discusses the need for occupation, and its association with well-being. Tessa Perrin defines what is meant by occupation and looks at ways to provide pleasurable activity. Achieving a balance between the cognitive capacity of a person and what they can meaningfully engage in, may involve the sensitive provision of age-inappropriate activities that are, however, pleasing and stimulating, as well as taking full advantage of sensory experiences.

The purpose of Part Four is to demonstrate the way that the 'problem behaviours' of aggression, wandering and confusion are now conceptualized as 'challenging behaviours', no longer constituting problems to be managed, but needs to be met. The result is that a new priority has emerged for practitioners and carers. In this section, Graham Stokes argues that the imperative is no longer to contain or control the behaviours that challenge us, but to resolve, by first establishing meaning and then pursuing potential solutions. Only when resolution is not possible do we consider how we and they may best cope.

In Part Five, 'Emotions and Therapeutic Interventions', we look at how we have become increasingly aware of the value of quality care cultures and how important it is to work with the feelings of those with dementia – people who are troubled and traumatised; denied a sense of emotional security by a combination of disease and dehumanisation. In Chapter 16, Ian Morton reviews the approaches that have sought to establish therapeutic relationships in dementia care and confront those aspects of caring that hinder the development of meaningful relationships. He critically appraises validation therapy, resolution therapy, pre-therapy and the work of Tom Kitwood and Dementia Care Mapping. Fiona Goudie then considers the nature of depression and emotional trauma in dementia, examining the potential for life review and psychological therapy to deliver true-therapeutic gains. In Chapter 19, John Wattis provides an up-to-date account of the role of psychotropic medication to calm distress and help to alleviate disturbed behaviour. In a significant development, the effectiveness of the so-called anti-dementia drugs (galantamine, donepizol and rivastagmine) is reviewed – a class of drug that was not even available a decade ago (who can say what the next 10 years hold?). In the final chapter, Marie Clare Shankland addresses the demands faced by family carers and how we may best work with those who can never go home and are always emotionally involved. By meeting the practical and emotional needs of caregivers, not only is their health and welfare respected, so is the well-being of their dependent loved ones.

As with *Working with Dementia*, this book can be read in its entirety, but the chapters are also written to stand alone, so the reader can select topics relevant to current interest.

We concluded the Preface to *Working with Dementia* with the hope that the horizons of dementia would be 'expanded through the application of creative thought to accepted theory and practice'. If the pace of change observed over the past 10 years characterises the next decade, then the perception of dementia as a *'silent* epidemic', provoking little interest and attracting only those who have failed elsewhere, will be irrevocably and thankfully assigned to history. We believe that over the lifetime of this book to work in dementia care will continue to be a journey through exciting and potentially radical times, jettisoning a lot that is accepted today, and acquiring much that is innovative and probably unexpected.

Graham Stokes
Fiona Goudie
August 2002

References

Benson S (ed), 2000, *Person-Centred Care*, Hawker Publications, London.
Cheston R & Bender M, 1999, *Understanding Dementia*, Jessica Kingsley, London.
Kitwood T, 1989, 'Brain, Mind and Dementia: With Particular Reference to Alzheimer's Disease', *Ageing and Society* 9, pp1–15.
Kitwood T, 1997, *Dementia Reconsidered*, Open University Press, London.
Kitwood T & Bredin K, 1992, *Person to Person*, Gale Centre Publications, Loughton.
Morton I, 1999, *Person-Centred Approaches to Dementia Care*, Speechmark Publishing/Winslow Press, Bicester.
Stokes G, 2000, *Challenging Behaviour in Dementia*, Speechmark Publishing/Winslow Press, Bicester.
Stokes G & Goudie F (eds), 1990, *Working with Dementia*, Speechmark Publishing/Winslow Press, Bicester.

PART 1

SETTING THE SCENE

CHAPTER 1

Attitudes to Dementia: A Decade of Change

Fiona Goudie

IN THE DECADE SINCE *WORKING WITH DEMENTIA* was published, there have been dramatic changes in public and professional attitudes to dementia and its treatment. Media attention has increased, aided by the 'coming out' of public figures such as the former US President Ronald Reagan and the author Iris Murdoch. A number of autobiographies and biographies have been published on the experience of Alzheimer's disease from the perspective of people with dementia (such as Robert Davis' account *My Journey into Alzheimer's Disease*) and their families (see, for example, Michael Ignatieff's *Scar Tissue*, Linda Grant's *Remind Me Who I Am Again*, and John Bailey's *Iris – A Memoir*). There is now a dedicated periodical – *Journal of Dementia Care* – an academic journal – *Dementia* – and the Alzheimer's Society has a national profile and an annual awareness week. The resulting improvements in public awareness mean that fewer people are likely to accept symptoms of dementia as part of the normal ageing process.

Attitudes to ageing are also changing as more people remain physically and mentally active into their late seventies and eighties, and expect healthcare to enable them to live high quality lives. There has been a rise in the number of centenarians in the UK, and in 1997 Jeanne Calment, aged 122 years, died in France of natural causes, having escaped cancer, cardiovascular disease and dementia. She lived independently until the age of 110. More medical and psychosocial research is being conducted into the effects of ageing. There are also dementia service development centres throughout the UK. Work in health- and social care with older people and people with dementia is now more likely to be seen as a positive career move than it was a decade ago.

Specific medical developments have taken place in the diagnosis and treatment of dementia, and new drugs are now available for the treatment of Alzheimer's disease. There is a need for a clear diagnosis before treatment can commence, and specialist memory clinics for early recognition of symptoms and diagnosis are becoming widely established. The emotional consequence of giving a diagnosis to people with dementia has presented a new challenge to many in the field of dementia care. Traditionally, carers may have been informed, but not people with dementia themselves. Research in other areas such as cancer, HIV/AIDS *and* among people with dementia has demonstrated the importance of considering the impact of diagnosis on the potential sufferer as well as their carers.

Practice developments in areas such as learning disability and neurological rehabilitation have generated interest. Advocacy for people with dementia to speak for themselves rather than have carers speak for them is a new development within dementia services, but it has a longer history in the learning disabilities field. So, too, has the right to a sexual identity. For the majority of people with dementia, issues of sexual expression will not be discussed unless public displays take place. Then medication becomes the most likely treatment option – to reduce the frequency of so-called sexual disinhibition, thus solving the problem for carers and other service users, but not necessarily for the person with dementia. In the field of neurological rehabilitation there has been an expansion in cognitive assessment and retraining strategies for people following stroke or head injury. Computer technology is increasingly used for assessment and rehabilitation programmes, addressing visuospatial and information-processing problems, as well as being used by people with communication difficulties. There have been some developments in computer-aided assessment for people with dementia, but so far only a few applications in treatment programmes such as computer-aided reality orientation or reminiscence packages.

There is a growing interest in the use of networked technology (the integration of cable technology, communications and information technology) to provide intelligent housing for the general population. A house could be designed with sensors enabling detection of open doors or windows; movements around the house (at night, for instance), or absence of movement by a certain time in the morning; overflow of bath or sink taps, and self-monitoring and adjustment of temperature control. This could mean more options for people with dementia to stay in their own home or to live in a sheltered community with such technology instead of moving to a residential or nursing home.

There has been an expansion in the use of conventional counselling and psychotherapy for people with dementia, in addition to specially developed approaches such as reminiscence, validation and resolution therapies. This has gone hand-in-hand with the change in emphasis to a person-centred approach and a 'new culture of dementia care' (Kitwood, 1997), and has not been restricted to people in the early stages of illness. Examples include individual counselling (Terry, 1997), cognitive-behaviour therapy (Teri & Gallagher Thompson, 1991), group therapy (Yale, 1995), and the use of stories in reminiscence (Cheston, 1996).

The centrality of carers and the importance of their needs has been formally acknowledged (Carers' [Recognition and Services] Act, 1995). Work with carers – the bedrock of service provision – continues to develop. More detailed work now exists on the nature of carer strain (Nolan, Grant & Keady, 1996), and on designing intervention programmes to provide the right sort of support when it is most needed. This is an area where research has identified that intervention can make a considerable impact on reducing carer distress and improving coping strategies.

The Law Commission (1995) has produced guidelines on decision-making for adults where mental capacity is impaired. These present a challenge to the usual practice in dementia care where decisions are taken by carers in the 'best interests' of the individual. Law Commission guidelines suggest that if an individual is unable currently to make their own decision, the principle of substituted judgement should be applied.

This involves making a decision based on what the person would want to do if they were able to speak up, and involves reviewing previous behaviour. It also involves the notion of 'the least restrictive alternative'. For example, a person may be able to make a decision about where they should live because they have the capacity to understand the options and implications, but not be able to manage their finances because of memory and calculation difficulties. Thus others may need to be involved in helping with finance, but not decisions about living circumstances. There are implications for assessment and care here – some have already been tested in the legal system – including the provision of locked wards, enduring power of attorney, and living wills.

Table 1.1 summarises some of the positive developments influencing good practice in dementia care.

Table 1.1 *Developments in dementia care*

- Growth in media profile
- Rising expectations of older population for healthcare
- Earlier diagnosis
- New drug treatments
- Transfer of ideas from fields of learning disabilities and neuro-rehabilitation
- Interest in computer and information technology applications
- Application of counselling and psychotherapy to dementia
- Potential of legislation for carers' needs
- Decision-making by people with dementia.

Challenges for change

The positive developments referred to above do not yet inform dementia services across the UK. There are a number of specific challenges summarised in Table 1.2 and discussed below.

Table 1.2 *Challenges for change*

- Cost of drugs could lead to competition between medical and psychological or social care.

- Fragmented public- and private-sector provision not geared to needs of people with dementia.

- Provision is poor for people with dementia from black and ethnic minority groups.

- Younger people with dementia have different symptoms and needs for support.

- Dominance of professionals in planning services and care.

- Social and demographic changes will mean fewer female middle-aged family carers to support older relatives.

- Ethical and legal issues associated with diagnosis and consent to treatment.

The cost of providing the new drugs for dementia

Drug costs and the associated services for diagnosing, monitoring and supporting people have not been fully funded by health authorities in the UK. Savings may be made by cutting back on existing services. This could lead to conflict between medical and psychosocial treatment and an unfortunate either/or scenario that is not supportive of the person-centred approach.

Fragmented provision

Despite the ageing of the population and the rise in expectations for high quality treatment, in reality services have been provided in an increasingly fragmented way. Political decisions throughout the 1980s and 1990s have meant that statutory organisations do not provide continuing health- and home care themselves, but negotiate the purchase of 'care packages' with the independent sector. Local authority guidance has restricted home care to people whose needs can be met within a given financial limit. This and the limited development of rehabilitation or convalescence models in independent sector homes have contributed to the rise in the number of people in permanent residential and nursing homes.

Needs of people from black and minority ethnic communities

The assessment and care needs of people from black and minority ethnic communities are still not adequately addressed. People with dementia in these communities are at risk of suffering from ignorance of religious and cultural experiences; misdiagnosis based on inappropriate assessment, and sometimes unchallenged racism from other service users and carers. Research has been undertaken to validate assessment instruments with Asian and African Caribbean communities (Rait *et al*, 2000a; Rait *et al*, 2000b). Further work is needed to increase the availability of translated material on dementia; make proper use of interpreters; develop outreach work through organisations already used by minority communities, and improve minority ethnic staffing levels in dementia services (Brownlie, 1991).

Provision for younger people with dementia

The numbers of younger people with dementia are small, and dedicated services appropriate to their age and needs are not widespread. Alzheimer's disease is less common. Pick's disease and other atypical dementias, where personality and subtle cognitive changes may occur before memory loss, is more likely. Assessment is less uniform and treatment has to focus on individual differences. A creative small-scale service has been developed for younger people with HIV-related dementia (de Villiers, 1997). Those campaigning for improvements in services for younger people have suggested schemes such as those provided by hospices as a good model for the continuing care needs of people with dementia. Lessons being learned about providing individualised services for younger people – rather than block provision of respite beds or day care, for example – can be applied to *all* people with dementia, on the basis that addressing difference and valuing diversity will improve services overall.

Dominance of professionals/carers in determining service delivery

Much of the planning of services, research, training and voluntary organisation activity has, until recently, been dominated by health- and social care 'professionals'. Voluntary organisations and campaign groups have been more inclusive, involving carers but rarely people with dementia themselves. There has been some change in this area. Goldsmith has published *Hearing the Voice of People with Dementia* (1996), and Rober Davis wrote of his developing dementia and crisis of religious faith. There are now a small number of advocacy schemes for people with dementia (Dunning, 1997). Just as services for people with learning disabilities and people with AIDS have changed because of the voice of service users, this is likely to occur with dementia. The conventional view has been that because people with dementia are mostly older, they are less challenging of service providers and less radical in expressing their views. This has not been universal and will continue to change as current cohorts of younger people age and are at risk of dementia.

Social changes reducing numbers of family carers

Currently two-thirds of carers are spouses and are older people themselves. The remainder are mostly daughters and daughters-in-law in middle age. Increases in separation and divorce; geographical mobility, and the number of women who work outside the home mean that this is likely to change. Furthermore, 'the declining numbers of descendants seem to be on a collision course with the surer survival of ageing kin' (Bengston & Treas 1980). It is not clear who the 'carers' of the twenty-first century will be.

Ethical and legal issues arising out of diagnosis

The availability of cognitive enhancers for Alzheimer's disease, combined with the increasing public awareness of dementia, is contributing to the increase in earlier assessment. Diagnosis of dementia may take place well before it becomes obvious to people outside a person's immediate family. There are ethical implications for work, driving, childcare and insurance associated with diagnosis. Services and service users have not traditionally had to address these issues or the associated ones of informed consent. For example, a person may have to inform their place of work or give up driving as a result of an early diagnosis sooner than if they had waited until the deterioration had been more evident to other people. There is much to be learned from the models of pre- and post-diagnostic counselling used in cancer, HIV and AIDS.

Summary
In the face of a potentially devastating disease, there is now the possibility of drug treatment that may reduce or delay the most negative symptoms of dementia. In many areas there are psychosocial and counselling services for people with dementia and their carers to help them cope with the consequences of the disease. Service providers in public, private and voluntary sectors continue to tackle ageism in general, and negative attitudes and low funding for dementia care in particular, in order to provide high quality care for people when they are most vulnerable. The changes in attitudes and developments in practice described in this chapter reflect the best current examples of dementia care. There is still much work to be done.

References

Bailey J, 1998, *Iris – A Memoir of Iris Murdoch,* Gerald Duckworth, London.

Bengston R & Treas, 1980, 'The changing family context of mental health and aging', in Birren JE & Sloane RB (eds), *Handbook of Mental Health and Aging*, Prentice Hall, Englewood Cliffs, New Jersey.

Brownlie J, 1991, *A Hidden Problem? Dementia amongst Ethnic Minority Groups*, Dementia Services Development Centre, University of Stirling.

Cheston R, 1996, 'Stories and metaphors: Talking about the past in a psychotherapy group for people with dementia', *Ageing & Society* 16, pp579–602.

Davis R, 1989, *My Journey into Alzheimer's Disease*, Scripture Press, Buckingham.

Department of Health, 1995, Carers (Recognition and Services) Act, Policy Guidance, London.

Dunning A, 1997 'Advocacy and Older People with Dementia', in Marshall M (ed), *State of the Art in Dementia Care*, Centre for Policy on Ageing, London.

Goldsmith M, 1996, *Hearing the Voice of People with Dementia: Opportunities and Obstacles,* Jessica Kingsley, London.

Grant L, 1998 *Remind me who I am Again*, Granta, London.

Ignatieff M, 1993, *Scar Tissue*, Chatto & Windus, London.

Kitwood T, 1997, *Dementia Reconsidered,* Open University Press, Buckingham.

Law Commission, 1995, *Mental Incapacity*, HMSO, London.

Nolan M, Grant G & Keady J, 1996, *'Understanding Family Care',* Open University Press, Buckingham.

Rait G, Burns A, Baldwin R, Chew-Graham C, Morley M & St Leger S, 2000a, 'Validating Screening Instruments for Cognitive Impairment in Older South Asians in the UK', *International Journal of Geriatric Psychiatry* 15, pp54–62.

Rait G, Morley M, Burns A, Baldwin R, Chew-Graham C & St Leger S, 2000b, 'Screening for Dementia in Older African-Caribbeans', *Psychological Medicine* 30, pp957–63.

Teri L & Gallagher-Thompson D, 1991, 'Cognitive-behavioural intervention for treatment of depression in Alzheimer's patients', *The Gerontologist* 31(3), pp413–16.

Terry P, 1997, *Counselling the Elderly and their Carers*, Macmillan, London.

De Villiers B, 1997, 'HIV-related dementia: the benefits of a small homely environment with a holistic client-centred approach', Marshall M (ed), *State of the Art in Dementia Care,* Centre for Policy on Ageing, London.

Yale R, 1995, *Developing Support Groups for Individuals with Early Stage Alzheimer's Disease: Planning, Implementation and Evaluation*, Health Professionals Press, Baltimore.

CHAPTER 2

The 'Dementias'

Una Holden & Graham Stokes

IN RECENT YEARS THERE HAVE BEEN enormous changes in knowledge and understanding with regard to 'dementia in old age', yet unfortunately antiquated beliefs about 'senile dementia' persist.

It is even possible that older people who exhibit signs of disorientation and strange behaviour may well be diagnosed as 'demented' when there is a much better explanation for their behaviour.

Case Study 2.1 Peter Parks' night-time behaviour

Peter Parks was 76 years old and was admitted into hospital because of his disturbing night-time behaviour. The staff were convinced that this previously mild-mannered man had something seriously wrong with his mind as every night he would become excessively restless, scream, shout and even howl. Anyone approaching him would be pushed away, or he would cower back and try to get underneath his bed. Was it dementia?

During the day he was sensible, rational and in control. When gently persuaded he eventually began to talk of his war-time experience in a Japanese prisoner of war camp. It soon became obvious that after holding back his horrendous experiences for so very many years, his tight control weakened at night and he relived some of the traumatic situations. By allowing himself to talk about his past he became more relaxed and more at peace.

So what is our contemporary understanding of dementia, and can it be accurately identified?

The causes of dementia

Untreatable brain diseases cause dementia – dementia being the name given to the syndromes that result from the brain pathology. Of the host of responsible diseases the most common are:

i) Alzheimer's disease (AD)

Named after Alois Alzheimer, the German physician who first identified this neurological disease of the cerebral cortex in 1907 (see Figure 2.1 for an illustration of the human cortex), Alzheimer's Disease (AD) is the most common form of dementia, accounting for at least 50 per cent of cases in later life. As with all presumptive diseases, definite diagnosis can only be determined after death.

AD sometimes appears in middle age (early onset dementia, EOD), but most often occurs after the age of 70 (late onset dementia, LOD).

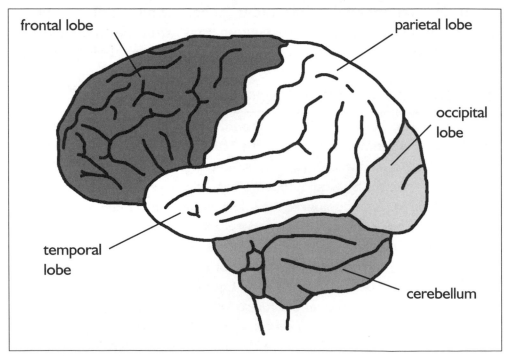

Figure 2.1 *The human cerebral cortex*

AD is progressive, irreversible, and pursues an unremitting course over a number of years. Dysfunction usually begins with mild memory problems, poor concentration, word-finding difficulties and impaired reasoning. These symptoms keep increasing in frequency and severity until memories are forgotten, disorientation reigns, and communication fails. Eventually, cognitive abilities are so severely impaired that the person becomes fully dependent on others.

While the current 'face' of dementia is AD, what is not widely appreciated is the fact that AD takes so many different forms that it probably does not really exist as a single disease entity (Cheston & Bender, 1999). One day, neuropathologists will have differentiated the cellular diseases that currently cluster under the umbrella of AD. A step in this direction occurred in the 1980s, with the identification of dementia with Lewy bodies.

ii)   Dementia with Lewy bodies (DLB)

Lewy bodies are degenerative lesions concentrated in the subcortical nuclei that have been recognised for many decades as among the important neuropathological changes in Parkinson's disease. In 1983 a Japanese research team discovered that these cells could be found in the cerebral cortex, and on such occasions were responsible for the onset of dementia (DLB). Two centres in the UK – Newcastle and Nottingham – investigated further and documented the typical signs and progressions of the disease (Byrne *et al*, 1989; McKeith *et al*, 1992). These are:

* Fluctuating dementia with lucid intervals
  a) Memory impairment
  b) Visuospatial deficits
  c) Disordered thought and reasoning
  d) Possible speech deficits.
* Clouding of consciousness, variable and episodic.
* Hallucinations, usually visual, some auditory. Often scenic. Worse at night.
* Paranoid delusions.
* Depression.

- Movement disorder typical of mild Parkinsonism. Possible falls.
- Neuroleptic sensitivity syndrome. The administration of neuroleptic (ie, anti-psychotic) medication can have adverse, at times fatal consequences (McKeith *et al*, 1992).

Recently, DLB has been pathologically confirmed in 15 per cent of cases of late-onset dementia (Holmes *et al*, 1999).

Case Story 2.2 Jessie's hallucinations

Jessie (68) lived alone and was very independent. She began to frighten her children by ringing them up, usually at night, screaming that someone was trying to get in to kill her. If she could not contact them she rang the police. On one occasion she berated her daughter for sitting down on an invisible (to the daughter) person. She was hospitalised for investigation. At times she was perfectly clear and sensible, even apologising for wasting the staff's time. Then suddenly she made no sense, did not recognise others, might fall over and had no idea of her whereabouts. She hallucinated. On one occasion she shouted at staff because they were doing nothing to save a child who was drowning somewhere on the other side of the room. Needless to say, there was no child and certainly no pool on the ward.

---

iii) Vascular dementia (VD)

The most common form of vascular dementia (VD) is multi-infarct dementia (MID), which follows a series of strokes, or infarcts, when a loss of blood flow damages specific areas of the brain. The stroke may be 'silent', being so small as to pass unnoticed. Hence the stroke is often referred to as a 'strokelet'. After several 'strokelets', sufficient brain tissue may be destroyed to result in dementia. MID accounts for about 20 per cent of dementia, and is generally observed in the seventh and eighth decades of life.

MID is a remitting dementia characterised by an abrupt onset. The course is typically that of a series of small strokes, which vary in frequency, intensity and location. They cause episodes of disorientation and loss of specific cognitive function. After the infarct there is usually limited clinical improvement until the next episode. As parts of the brain may be spared, or are yet to be affected by stroke, the cognitive picture is patchy and inconsistent. Eventually, after a succession of infarcts, there is less and less recovery, until by a process of 'stepwise' deterioration, dementia as widespread as AD develops.

Early onset dementia (EOD)

A phenomenon of the 1990s has been an increasing awareness of the prevalence of dementia in middle age (referred to as either early onset dementia [EOD] or younger onset dementia [YOD]). Harvey (1998) estimates there are approximately 17,000 people in the UK below the age of 65 years with dementia. The syndrome is associated with heterogeneous pathology; the appearance of non-cognitive signs (for example, hallucinations and delusions); carer strain, and a consequent demand for institutional care. While the diseases are largely the same as those observed in later life, Table 2.1 illustrates that the pattern of EOD is, however, different (Harvey, 1998).

Table 2.1 The pattern of early onset dementia (EOD)

	% of cases
Alzheimer's disease	34
Dementia with Lewy bodies	7
Vascular dementia	18
Fronto-temporal dementia	12
Alcohol-related dementia	10
Other (eg, Huntington's disease, multiple sclerosis, Down's syndrome)	19

Table 2.1 shows that pathology rarely encountered in old age is more commonly seen among younger people. For example, alcohol-related dementia is the result of chronic alcohol dependency, and is most often diagnosed in early middle age, while fronto-temporal dementia may be a true EOD.

Fronto-temporal dementia (FTD)

Fronto-temporal dementia (FTD – also known as frontal lobe dementia) has attracted significant clinical attention only since the 1980s (eg, Gustafson, 1987; Hodgson & Barrett, 1993).

This dementia is associated with cellular disease of the frontal and temporal lobes of the cerebral cortex. A family history occurs in almost half the cases. In a minority of cases, FTD involves cellular degeneration known as Pick's disease – a cerebral pathology first described at the beginning of the last century (Pick, 1906). While FTD is observed as both an early and late onset syndrome, far more cases are seen in middle age. In later life, FTD is considered rare (Harvey 1998).

The most common clinical features of FTD are:

- Personality changes
  a) Apathy, indifference OR disinhibition and restlessness
  b) Stereotyped behaviour – perseveration, rituals and food fads
  c) No insight or empathy for others
  d) Loss of social awareness
  e) Neglect of responsibilities
- Sterile speech, echolalia, eventually mutism
- Poor judgement and impaired reasoning.
- Problems of verbal fluency and production
- Early onset incontinence
- No neurological signs.

As years pass and the disease progresses, FTD conforms to the classical picture of Alzheimer's disease.

Uncommon dementias

Aside from the frequently encountered diseases that cause dementia, there are many other less common dementia syndromes.

Creutzfeldt-Jakob disease (CJD)

Creutzfeldt-Jakob disease (CJD) is a rare condition. There are fears, however, that it will become more common in the UK and mainland

---

Case Study 2.3 Maggie's changing behaviour

Maggie (64) attends the day hospital, and both staff and relatives are puzzled by her behaviour. Once an outgoing, lively woman she now has a fixed stare and stiff walk. She wanders about the unit or her home counting things, picking them up and rearranging them in lines. Every so often she repeats what she or others say and some people are insulted when she copies their gestures. A major difficulty is her eating behaviour, as one day she will gobble everything placed in front of her and the next day refuse the food that she liked the day before.

Europe because of its association with Bovine Spongiform Encephalopathy (BSE) (first identified in 1995 and known as variant CJD). Whether this will occur, only time will tell. Currently, the prevalence rate in the UK is estimated to be just one case per million people.

CJD was first described in the 1920s. Both an inherited and transmissible condition, it causes a progressive loss of cognitive abilities and is accompanied by neurological symptoms such as unsteadiness and clumsiness. Most cases (85 per cent) are sporadic, having no known cause, with the remainder comprising familial, iatrogenic and variant. The peak age of onset of sporadic CJD is between 60 and 65 years. Young people are affected by variant CJD (average age is 28 years).

Early symptoms often resemble depression – low mood, poor memory, social withdrawal and disinterest. However, rapid progression to dementia and obvious neurological symptoms distinguish CJD from depression. Within weeks, the person may become unsteady on their feet, lacking in coordination and markedly clumsy. Later symptoms include visual impairment, rigidity, jerky movements, speech deficits and incontinence. Eventually, the person loses the ability to move or speak.

Seventy per cent of people die within six months of the symptoms appearing. Rarely, CJD lasts for several years. The course of variant CJD is typically around two years.

Case Study 2.4 Colin's rapid deterioration

Colin (41) started to arrive home late from work, offering his wife the lamest of excuses. He hadn't been able to find his car keys; he couldn't locate his car; he had forgotten the route home. His wife, disbelieving, thought he was having an affair – a suspicion heightened by his lack of interest in her and their home. Then she started to notice out of character failings. Nothing major, but puzzling all the same. Colin would not always flush the toilet; he would often forget to put the cap back on the toothpaste. Colin himself was worried. His family doctor diagnosed stress.

Colin deteriorated rapidly. Not only did he become more forgetful, but his coordination was poor, his balance was unsteady and he became irrationally fearful of intruders. By now it was clear that he was dementing dramatically. He suffered from hallucinations and would become agitated and distressed. Colin could not tolerate noise or bright light. As his dementia became profound, his wife could no longer cope and he entered a nursing home, where he now lies in a state of total dependency, seemingly unresponsive to all around him. Less than two years has elapsed since this wife first thought Colin was concealing an extra-marital affair.

AIDS dementia complex (ADC)

There has always been a sexually transmitted dementia. Traditionally it was the consequence of syphilis, and was known as the grand paralysis of the insane (GPI). Nowadays, this is rarely seen. We now encounter dementia that is the product of HIV (ADC is also known as HIV-associated dementia). The early signs are:

- Exaggerated forgetfulness
- Loss of concentration
- Slowness of thought and movement
- Loss of balance
- Motor impairments
- Apathy and social withdrawal.

Later developments include:

* Gross cognitive dysfunction
* Incontinence
* Mutism
* Paralysis.

The prevalence of dementia in people with AIDS is between 8 and 16 per cent (Catalan & Burgess, 1996). Dementia typically develops over a relatively short period of time – usually a few months. Once present, dementia is associated with poor prognosis. Median life expectancy may be as brief as six months, during which time challenging behaviour and mood disturbance may be observed.

In recent times, several unusual conditions have appeared. These remain poorly accepted and, in the most part, ignored. An example is organophosphate poisoning, which may occur following exposure and can affect people regardless of age.

Organophosphate is found in certain insecticide sprays used, for instance, against warble fly, in sheep dip and in certain pesticides. Certain areas of the UK have reported cases, of all ages, suffering from the effects. They include:

* Memory loss
* Inattention
* Symptoms typical of myalgia encephalomyelitis (ME)
* Language disorder
* Sudden vacancies – ie, pauses in thinking, writing and conversation
* Anxiety and restlessness (early symptoms)
* Depression.

Physical signs include:

* Headache, nausea and dizziness (early symptoms)
* Muscle twitching, tremor, poor coordination, nausea, diarrhoea and stomach cramps

- Sweating, rhinorrhea, salivation, coughing and tears
- MIOSIS – contraction of the eyes, blurred vision (Holden, 1996)

Various other syndromes, such as progressive fluent aphasia (Kirschner *et al*, 1987); semantic dementia (Hodges *et al*, 1992), and progressive posterior cortical atrophy (Victoroff *et al*, 1994) have been identified, as well as a number of vascular conditions aside from MID, including Binswanger's disease (Peretz & Cummings, 1988) and CADASIL (Martin & Markus, 2001). There is also the syndrome of subcortical dementia caused by cellular pathology – for example, Parkinson's disease and progressive supranuclear palsy (Peretz & Cummings, 1988).

In the near future it is likely that many more 'new' diseases will be identified, and new ways to work with both the people affected and their families will be required. It is vital, therefore, that care staff are always aware of developments, and work to ensure that a true diagnosis is given, rather than being satisfied with 'they've got dementia'.

References

Byrne EJ, Lennox G, Low J & Goodwin-Austen RB, 1989, 'Diffuse Lewy Body Disease, Clinical Features in 15 Cases', *Journal of Neurology, Neurosurgery and Psychiatry* 5, pp709–17.

Catalan J & Burgess A, 1996, 'HIV-associated dementia and related disorders', *International Review of Psychiatry,* 8, pp237–43.

Cheston & Bender, 1999, *Understanding Dementia*, Jessica Kingsley, London.

Gustafson, L, 1987, 'Frontal lobe degeneration of non-Alzheimer type 11, Clinical picture and differential diagnosis', *Archives of Gerontological Geriatrics* 6, pp209–23.

Harvey RJ, 1998, *Young Onset Dementia*, Imperial College School of Medicine, London.

Hodges JR, Patterson K, Oxbury S & Funnell E, 1992, 'Semantic Dementia', *Brain* 115, pp1783–806.

Hodgson RE & Barrett K, 1993, 'Dementia of Frontal Lobe Type in Monozygotic Twins', *International Journal of Geriatric Psychiatry* 8, pp431–4.

Holden UP, 1996, 'Dipping into a Poisonous Problem', *Journal of Dementia Care,* May/June, pp10–11.

Holmes C, Cairns N, Lantos P & Mann A, 1999, 'Validity of Current Clinical Criteria for Alzheimer's disease, Vascular Dementia and Dementia with Lewy Bodies', *British Journal of Psychiatry* 174, pp45–50.

Kirschner HS, Tanridag O, Thurman L & Whetsell WO, 1987, 'Progressive aphasia without dementia: two cases with spongiform degeneration', *Annals of Neurology* 22, pp527–32.

Martin R & Markus H, 2001, 'CADASIL: a genetic form of subcortical vascular dementia', *Dementia Reviews* 4(1), pp1–6.

McKeith I, Fairbairn A, Perry R, Thompson P & Perry E, 1992, 'Neuroleptic Sensitivity in Patients with Senile Dementia of Lewy Body Type', *British Medical Journal* 305, pp673–8.

Peretz JA & Cummings JL, 1988, 'Subcortical Dementia', in Holden UP (ed), *Neuropsychology and Ageing,* Croom Helm, London.

Pick A, 1906, 'Uber einen weiterer Symptomenkomplex im Rahmen der Dementia senilis, bedingt durch unschriebene starkere Hirnatrophie (gemishche Apraxie)', *Monatschrift for Psychiatrie und Neurologie* 19, pp97–108.

Ryan C & Butters N, 1986, 'Neuropsychology of alcoholism', in Wedding D, Horton AM Jr. & Webster JS (eds), *The Neuropsychology Handbook,* Springer, New York.

Victoroff J, Webster Ross G, Benson F, Verity A & Vinters HV, 1994, 'Posterior cortical atrophy', *Archives Neurology* 51(March), pp269–74.

Further reading

Byrne EJ, 1987, 'Reversible dementia', *International Journal of Geriatric Psychiatry* 2, pp73–81.

Cox S & Keady J, 1999, *Younger People with Dementia*, Jessica Kingsley, London.

Holden UP, 1995, *Ageing, Neuropsychology and the New 'Dementias'*, Chapman & Hall, London.

CHAPTER 3

Physical and Emotional Problems in Later Life

Fiona Goudie

SOME PHYSICAL AND EMOTIONAL PROBLEMS are responsible for cognitive and memory problems in older people. They may be mistaken for dementia, but if properly identified may respond to treatment so that the memory and cognitive problems are reduced or removed.

This chapter examines some of these conditions; the similarities and differences between them and dementia, and discusses implications for treatment.

Physical problems

Certain chronic conditions such as cardiovascular disease and hypertension are associated with mildly impaired cognitive functioning. Sensory deficits such as visual and hearing impairment may affect orientation and communication – particularly in unfamiliar settings. Medication for specific problems may also impair functioning. These can contribute to misdiagnosis of dementia in older people. Some of the specific physical problems that can be mistaken for dementia in older people are discussed more fully in this section.

Delirium (acute confusional state)

Delerium may be mistaken for dementia in older people – especially if the older person is in hospital, or is being assessed by someone who has not known them prior to the onset of the acute confusion. Delirium is not a specific illness, but results from a change in the body's metabolism, which can lead to high temperature, fever and disturbance of consciousness. This in turn can bring about temporary disorientation; memory loss; a state of 'muddled perplexity'; poor concentration; hallucinations; clouding of consciousness, and restlessness. It is often worse at night.

The changes in metabolism can be due to a number of factors. Some of these are listed in Table 3.1. The acute confusion usually arises fairly suddenly – over a few hours or days with an acute infection – although it may take weeks or months for rarer metabolic problems, such as chronic liver disease. It will disappear if the underlying condition can be treated. People with dementia and chronic physical health problems are particularly susceptible to acute confusion. For them, the underlying dementia will not vanish when the cause of the acute confusion is treated, but the sudden, recent symptoms will.

Table 3.1 *Causes of delirium*

- Chest and urinary tract infections
- Vitamin B_{12} deficiency (associated with severe anaemia)
- Thiamine deficiency (associated with poor diet or alcohol misuse)
- Endocrine disturbances, such as diabetes or thyroid deficiency
- Drugs (especially hypnotics, some Parkinsonian drugs and antidepressants)
- Excess alcohol consumption
- Heart, kidney, liver or respiratory disease
- Dehydration
- Stroke, transient ischaemic attacks (TIAs) or head injury
- Constipation
- Hypothermia
- Trauma following surgery or a fracture
- Sleep disturbance
- Environmental changes, such as moving house or going into hospital
- Depression and bereavement reactions.

Parkinson's disease

Parkinson's disease occurs as a result of cell loss in the basal ganglia, an area in the underlying structure of the brain. Microscopic structures called Lewy bodies form in the remaining cells. Cell loss severely reduces the production of a neurotransmitter called dopamine, leading to characteristic physical symptoms. The main ones are tremor, muscular rigidity, slowness of movement (bradykinesia) and postural problems. Additional problems include excessive salivation, urinary disturbance, tiredness, slowed thought processes (bradyphrenia) and depression. One or two people per thousand will be affected. Two-thirds of people with Parkinson's disease have the first signs between the ages of 50 and 69 years.

The term Parkinsonism is used to describe the clinical syndrome (tremor, muscular rigidity, bradykinesis and postural abnormality) when dopamine deficiency is present, but there is no cell loss. It can occur as a result of boxing-related head injury, anoxia following cardiac arrest, or carbon monoxide poisoning. It can also be drug-induced. In this case, the symptoms disappear over several weeks once the drug is stopped.

Misdiagnosis can occur in the early stages. Slowness of movement may be attributed to depression or thyroid deficiency; limb rigidity and pain may be explained as arthritis. Depression occurs in about two-fifths of sufferers, and is likely to be a combination of physical (biochemical imbalance), psychological (impact of the illlness) and social factors (effects on work and social activities). Depression added to motor slowness may result in poor performance on behavioural and cognitive assessments, and a misdiagnosis of dementia may be given. Oyebode *et al* (1986) found that few of the cognitive problems in Parkinson's disease were consistent with those found in Alzheimer's disease. However, the picture is complex as in the later stages a proportion of people will develop dementia. Peretz and Cummings (1988) believe this is a subcortical dementia, whereas Knight *et al* (1988) consider the cognitive changes to be part of early Alzheimer's disease.

Dementia is more likely when the onset of Parkinson's disease is later in life (after 70 years of age), and less likely if it started before the age of 50.

Parkinsonian symptoms of tremor and rigidity are reduced by drug treatment. Levodopa (Sinemet or Madopar) is the treatment of choice.

Effectiveness may be reduced after a period of about five years. Side-effects such as agitation, hallucinations and delusions can occur. These are more likely with long-term use, so careful monitoring of medication is important.

Input from a multidisciplinary rehabilitation team is key to the management of Parkinson's disease. This will involve the monitoring of drugs by the medical team; physiotherapy for managing stiffness, gait and mobility problems; occupational therapy to help devise rehabilitation strategies to make the most of preserved physical abilities, minimise fatigue and advise on aids and adaptations in the home; and speech and language therapy for difficulties with weak muscles, which may result in dysarthria and poor voice projection. Emotional support for the individual and their family will be available from members of such a team, which will include nurses and possibly a psychologist. Long-term support groups may be linked to a rehabilitation team or voluntary agency (Parkinson's Disease Society).

Stroke

A cerebrovascular accident (CVA) or 'stroke' occurs as a result of an infarction in the blood vessels to and within the brain, or a haemorrhage in the brain. About five in every 1,000 people over 65 years old are affected by stroke, although a quarter of all people with strokes are under 65 years of age. Onset is usually sudden. Symptoms vary depending on the site of the stroke, but the most common are: changes in muscle tone resulting in limb weakness or paralysis; speech and language impairment; visual and perceptual difficulties; cognitive, personality and emotional changes.

Limb weakness or paralysis and language impairments are usually the most obvious, and are the focus of early rehabilitation. However, certain cognitive deficits may be subtle. Difficulties with vision, perception, memory, planning and problem-solving will affect physical rehabilitation, and in the absence of skilled assessment, may be misdiagnosed as dementia. See the following case study for an illustration of this.

Transient ischaemic attacks (TIAs) are small strokes that affect specific aspects of cognitive functioning. At first the person will recover from the effects of the TIA within hours or days. However, as the attacks increase in number the residual damage is not reversible, and a picture of

Case Study 3.1 Mr Young's stroke

Mr Young was a 69-year-old widower who had moved to a new town to live near his sister. He had fallen over while shopping in the town centre and appeared dishevelled and confused. He was admitted to hospital for an assessment.

He appeared to make a rapid physical recovery. However, he had difficulty orientating himself on the ward, and did not appear to recognise staff even after several days' stay. During the kitchen assessment conducted by the occupational therapist, he tried to pour water into the toaster rather than the kettle and use bowls rather than cups for tea. A further assessment by the clinical psychologist revealed that Mr Young had some specific perceptual problems (he could not recognise familiar objects or faces) and difficulty judging space and distance, which made him clumsy. He had visual memory problems because of these difficulties, which explained why he could not recognise staff. His verbal memory was unaffected and he could remember information he had been told or had written down. A CT scan of his brain showed a specific stroke in the cortical area responsible for visual perception. He was not dementing and benefitted from a period of rehabilitation aimed at building up his confidence by using verbal lists and labels and checking street and shop names rather than relying on landmarks that he found hard to recognise.

vascular dementia emerges (see Chapter 2). TIAs affect cortical and subcortical areas of the brain, leading to patchy cognitive functioning and abilities that vary from day to day, often worsening in the evenings.

Head injury
Although head injuries affect larger numbers of younger people, falls and related head injuries are more common in older people. Head injury after a fall may go undiagnosed and specific, non-progressive, cognitive deficits may be wrongly attributed to dementia. Psychological problems associated with post-traumatic stress following the injury include anxiety, depression and phobic reactions. These can affect concentration, memory and problem-

solving abilities. There is some evidence that head injury in later life results in dementia more frequently than at a younger age (Holden, 1988).

Subdural haematoma is a type of tumour that can lead to dramatic cognitive problems affecting memory, visuospatial abilities and language. Surgery to remove the haematoma can be successful regardless of the age of the individual, and many abilities can be partly or completely restored.

Age-associated memory impairment

This is a new category of memory impairment, which is considered to be more serious than the effects of normal ageing, but not as significant as dementia. It is not thought to be progressive. It is a controversial clinical category, and more research is needed to ensure that it differs significantly from the effects of depression or anxiety in normal ageing, non-progressive injury, or a very slowly progressing and hard-to-measure condition.

Emotional problems

The onset of dementia is often accompanied by depression and anxiety. However, at times, the extent of psychological distress can be so severe that it may be misinterpreted as dementia. There are also certain other psychological and psychiatric problems (including mania, hallucinations, delusions, paraphrenia and alcohol misuse) associated with confusion and impaired cognitive functioning. These are discussed in the next section.

Depression

Depression is the most common emotional problem affecting older people, and is often undiagnosed. Certain groups of people are particularly vulnerable to depression, including those with physical illness, people in residential and nursing homes, and family caregivers. Symptoms of depression include pervasive low mood; poor memory and concentration; appetite and sleep disturbance; loss of interest in life; preoccupation with physical complaints; agitation or retardation of movement, and feelings of worthlessness. Thoughts of death or suicide may also feature.

Even when depression has been properly identified, large numbers of older people do not receive treatment or referral to specialist services

(McDonald, 1986). This may be because depression is considered normal or inevitable in older people, or because drug or psychological treatments most suited to older people are not offered. If it is left untreated, depression can become severe, and some symptoms may mimic dementia. Self-neglect associated with poor appetite and sleep disturbance; apathetic withdrawal leading to social avoidance; poor concentration and slowed thought processes may all lead to a misdiagnosis. Table 3.2 summarises some of the differences between depression and Alzheimer's disease.

Severe depression can result in profound psychomotor retardation or agitation and apparent cognitive impairment, which improves as the depression is treated. This syndrome may be termed 'depressive pseudodementia'. However, it is a rather misleading term as people with cognitive impairment during a depressive episode are more likely to develop dementia in the future, even if they respond well to treatment initially.

Table 3.2 *Differences between depression and Alzheimer's disease*

The person with depression	The person with Alzheimer's
Often complains of poor memory.	May be unaware of memory problems.
May say 'I don't know' in answer to questions requiring concentration.	May confabulate or make up answers to questions requiring good concentration or memory. May appear unaware that answer is wrong.
Has fluctuating ability and uneven impairment on cognitive testing.	Tends to show consistent global impairment on cognitive testing.
Gives up easily, poorly motivated.	Has a go.
May be slow but successful in complex tasks, aware of errors.	Has problems with complex tasks involving concentration. Often unaware of errors.

Chapter 17 discusses psychological interventions for depression in more detail, and Chapter 19 describes antidepressant medication.

Mania and hypomania

Overactivity without cognitive impairment is the main clinical feature of mania. The person may be excessively elated or irritable, with grandiose ideas and delusions (persistent false beliefs). Hypomania is a milder form of mania, and the terms may be used interchangeably. Some forms of frontal lobe dementia characterised by disinhibited behaviour can mimic mania. It may be difficult to assess the person with mania as they may be unwilling to cooperate with formal testing. Drug treatment in the context of ongoing community support for the person and their family is likely to be successful, although compliance is often problematic among people with mania.

Anxiety

Anxiety is more common than depression in older people. The physical manifestations of unrealistic or excessive worry (such as palpitations; sweating; butterflies in the stomach; feelings of sickness or diarrhoea) can be wrongly attributed to physical illness by older people themselves, and by their carers. Acute anxiety can lead to panic attacks and hyperventilation (breathing at an abnormally fast rate, which induces dizziness, faintness, tightening chest, tingling fingers and toes, aches and pains), which can impair concentration and the ability to carry out routine tasks. The fear of the symptoms (which may be misinterpreted as a heart attack) can result in the person avoiding the situation they believed brought them on in the first place (phobic avoidance).

Panic attacks may be part of a phobic disorder. The most common of these in older people is agoraphobia (manifest as fear of leaving the house; of social situations; of shopping and using public transport), which can result in crippling social withdrawal and isolation. Anxiety and social withdrawal are relatively common in the early phases of dementia, as the individual tries to avoid exposure to stressful activities and public embarrassment.

Relaxation training, which teaches how to relax the body and mind and control erratic breathing, can be incorporated into an anxiety-management programme. This will focus on helping the person cope with the specific triggers for their own anxiety (see Chapter 17). Hyperventilation (Holden,

1988) suggests that this occurs when someone breathes at a rate of more than 20 breaths per minute in the absence of an alternative medical reason) can be helped by strategies that teach breathing from the diaphragm rather than the thorax, and encourage the person to slow down their rate of breathing.

'Free floating anxiety' describes a state for which there is no obvious trigger. It can be more difficult to treat because the person cannot readily learn strategies to cope with fearful situations. However, relaxation exercises and techniques for dealing with hyperventilation can help. Anxiety frequently coexists with depression and may respond well to treatment with antidepressants.

As a rule, benzodiazepines (tranquillisers and hypnotics) are recommended for short-term use only as the effect wears off after a few weeks and withdrawal effects can be marked. Unfortunately, long-term benzodiazepine use is common among older people, and is linked with falls and confusion. The relaxation training and anxiety-management techniques described above can be used to help people withdraw from benzodiazepines, and may also help with sleeping problems.

Hallucinations, delusions and paraphrenia

Auditory hallucinations are found most commonly in schizophrenia, although they can occur in severe depression. They may be present in paraphrenia (see below). Visual hallucinations are frequently associated with acute confusional states and alcohol or drug withdrawal (delirium tremens). They can also occur in vascular or dementia with Lewy bodies. Hallucinations of touch and smell are rare in older people, although people who have had a stroke may experience hallucinatory sensations of touch or movement in one of their affected limbs.

Delusions are persistent false beliefs incompatible with the individual's cultural and educational background (Wattis & Martin, 1994). They can occur in delirium or in severe depression. Examples include delusions of an incurable illness, or that the person has committed a terrible crime. The drug treatment for delusions is similar to that used in schizophrenia.

Late paraphrenia (or paranoid schizophrenia in old age) occurs in less than one per cent of those over the age of 65 years. The syndrome is viewed as a late-onset disorder with 'a well organised system of paranoid delusions with or without auditory hallucinations in the setting of a well preserved personality and affective response' (Roth, 1955). The condition seems to be most common among socially isolated women, with few family links, who are deaf and live in inadequate housing.

Individuals may have delusions about being persecuted, spied on or attacked. Calling on neighbours and the police may trigger awareness among others of the disorder. In some instances paraphrenic symptoms may be associated with non-progressive organic changes in the brain and mildly impaired cognitive functioning (Hymas *et al*, 1989). Neuroleptic medication is the treatment of choice – often given as a depot injection. Some success has been reported with behavioural interventions (Carstensen & Fremouw, 1981).

Family, friends and home carers have an important role to play in supporting the individual diagnosed with any of these conditions. The input over time from members of a community mental health team will be invaluable. A person-centred approach that acknowledges feelings rather than confronting inaccurate statements head on is likely to be the most productive. It is important to be aware that moving house is unlikely to solve the problem of auditory hallucinations as the 'voice' is likely to move too.

Alcohol misuse

Alcohol misuse is a significant mental health problem in later life. While the number of older people who drink regularly declines with age, about a fifth of male and female drinkers consume more than the recommended safe limits for alcohol intake.

While alcohol abuse can be part of a long-term pattern, there are some people who develop alcohol problems for the first time. This may be part of a strategy to cope with loneliness, bereavement and social isolation. Drinking can also be used as a pain relief strategy. Denial can make it difficult to identify the problem and underlying causes.

Metabolic changes in later life mean alcohol can have a more profound effect on attention, concentration and general cognition than it would have at a younger age. If heavy drinking is associated with poor eating habits, confusion can be marked. Long-term use may be associated with the irreversible symptoms of alcohol-related dementia and Korsakoff's syndrome. However, if the alcohol misuse has developed recently, treatment aimed at the underlying problem (bereavement, loneliness, pain and so on) can help a planned withdrawal and relieve the cognitive problems.

Conclusions

This chapter does not cover all the conditions that may be mistaken for dementia, but attempts to emphasise the importance of excluding other conditions rather than jumping to the conclusion that dementia is present.

It is important that those involved in assessing and supporting people with dementia can differentiate dementia from other physical, psychiatric or psychological problems. They require different treatments and may result in the reduction or removal of some of the distressing cognitive, psychological and social problems that can occur independently or may coexist with dementia.

References

Carstensen LL & Fremouw WJ, 1981, 'The Demonstration of a Behavioural Intervention for Late Life Paranoia', *Gerontologist* 21, pp329–33.

Holden U, 1988, 'Head Injury and Older People,' in U Holden (ed), *Neuropsychology and Ageing*, Croom Helm, London, pp154–76.

Hymas N, Naguib M & Levy R, 1989, 'Late Paraphrenia: a follow-up study', *International Journal of Geriatric Psychiatry* 4, pp23–9.

Knight RG, Godfrey HPD, & Shelton EJM, 1988, 'The psychological deficits associated with Parkinson's disease', *Clinical Psychology Review* 8, pp391–410.

McDonald AJD, 1986, 'Do General Practitioners "miss" Depression in Elderly Patients?', *British Medical Journal* 292, 24 May, pp1365–7.

Oyebode J, Barker WA, Blessed G, Dick DJ & Britton PG, 1986, 'Cognitive functioning in Parkinson's Disease', *British Journal of Psychiatry* 149, pp720–5.

Peretz JA & Cummings JL, 1988, 'Subcortical dementia', in Holden UP (ed), *Neuropsychology and Ageing*, Croom Helm, London.

Roth M, 1955, 'The natural history of mental disorder in old age', *Journal of Mental Science* 101, pp281–301.

Wattis J & Martin C, 1994, *Practical Psychiatry of Old Age*, 2nd edn, Chapman & Hall, London.

PART 2
DISCOVERY

CHAPTER 4

Cognitive and Behavioural Assessment

Fiona Goudie

Introduction

Growing awareness of the existence of dementia syndromes and new treatment possibilities has led to an increase in demand for cognitive assessment to:

- Inform diagnosis
- Provide information to clients on strengths and difficulties
- Assess the impact of drug and psychological interventions
- Monitor change over time
- Support assessment of functional abilities, such as driving.

Assessment of behaviour and activities of daily living (ADL) has developed beyond using rating scales to determine whether or not someone can perform self-care tasks like feeding and toileting to encompass the more individualised approach outlined by Stokes in this book. New scales have been developed, which aim to assess why a person can or cannot do a given task, and which can be used as a basis for treatment and rehabilitation. There are also new assessment measures of mood and challenging behaviour. The development in person-centred approaches means that the quality of life of the person with dementia is valued, and consideration is increasingly being given as to how to evaluate this – particularly among people who may not be able to speak for themselves.

This chapter outlines some of these assessment tools and considers when they should be used. Case examples are given to illustrate the purpose of some of the different kinds of assessment.

Cognitive assessment

Cognitive assessment of memory and intellectual ability is an essential element of assessment for diagnosis, as well as providing a baseline against which change as a result of intervention can be measured. Strengths and weaknesses may be highlighted and strategies developed to address these.

The cognitive deficits most commonly found in dementia of the Alzheimer's type are memory impairment; aphasia (language impairment); apraxia (disorders of coordination); agnosia (disorders of recognition), and disturbance in executive functioning (such as planning, organising, sequencing and abstracting). In order to reach a diagnosis, a cognitive assessment should examine all these abilities. It will be used along with the medical assessment and history from the person and from someone who knows them well.

A number of well validated screening tools to detect possible impairment exist. They include the Abbreviated Mental Test (AMT – Hodkinson, 1972); Information/Orientation section of the Clifton Assessment Procedure for the Elderly (CAPE – Pattie & Gilleard, 1979), and the Mini Mental State Examination (MMSE – Folstein *et al*, 1975). These can be used by general practitioners, health professionals and social work staff as a preliminary assessment, but are not sufficient to provide a diagnosis of dementia on their own, although they may reveal problems with memory, orientation and verbal expression that might be due to dementia or another health problem. Work has been undertaken with the AMT and MMSE to validate them for use with Asian and African Caribbean older people (Rait *et al*, 2000a; 2000b).

More detailed assessments might be used by psychologists or trained staff in a community mental health team or memory clinic. Examples include the Cognitive Examination from the Cambridge Assessment of Mental Disorders in the Elderly (CAMDEX; Roth *et al*, 1988); Alzheimer's

Disease Assessment Scale Cognitive Subscale (ADAS-COG; Rosen *et al*, 1984), or the computerised Cambridge Neuropsychological Automated Test Battery (CANTAB; Sahakian, 1990). These examine a range of cognitive functions known to be impaired in dementia; not only memory and orientation, but also language, speed of information processing, abstract reasoning and psychomotor skills.

Behavioural assessment and assessment of activities of daily living (ADLs)

The ability to communicate, mobilise and undertake self-care tasks, such as bathing, toileting and feeding (Activities of Daily Living, or ADLs), along with the presence of behaviour problems, may be rated using scales like the CAPE Behaviour Rating Scale (Pattie & Gilleard, 1979), or Behavioural Assessment Scale of Later Life (BASOLL; Brooker, 1997). Instrumental Activities of Daily Living (IADLs) encompass tasks that require more complex planning and problem-solving, such as shopping, cooking and organising transport. Such scales are usually completed by a carer, and rate whether or not someone can perform a particular task successfully and how much support they need. Examples include the Instrumental Activities of Daily Living Scale (Lawton & Brody, 1969); Bristol Activities of Daily Living Scale (Bucks *et al*, 1996), and Nurses' Observation Scale for Geriatric Patients (Spiegel *et al*, 1991).

Some IADL scales place greater emphasis on the *process* of performing an activity – how it is done – rather than how successfully it has been performed. Process involves attention, organisation, planning and motor ability. The individual is observed carrying out a task, such as dressing or making a phone call, and their competence is analysed. For instance, did they have a problem putting steps of the task in order; did they seem to miss out a step or have difficulty with motor co-ordination? Such assessment can be used as a basis for treatment-planning in rehabilitation and retraining. Examples of scales that focus on process include the Kitchen Task Assessment (Baum & Edwards, 1993) and the Functional Performance Measure (Carswell *et al*, 1995).

There are now some standardised rating scales specifically designed to measure disturbed mood and challenging behaviour associated with dementia – for example, the Revised Memory and Behaviour Problems

Checklist, Teri *et al*, 1992; Rating Scale for Aggressive Behaviour (RAGE), Patel & Hope, 1992; Present Behavioural Examination (PBE), Hope & Fairburn, 1992.

Diagnosis

Cognitive and behavioural assessments contribute to the diagnosis of dementia, together with physical, psychiatric and neurological tests (including relevant brain scans), and the history from the individual and their family or friends.

A short cognitive assessment using the MMSE, for example, may be sufficient if there is a clear history of progressive decline in IADLs over a couple of years, and there is no alternative explanation for the changes – medical or otherwise. The MMSE has a maximum score of 30. The questions cover orientation to time and place (for example, day, date and address); memory (recalling the names of three objects); attention (for example, serial subtraction of 7 from 100); language (such as naming objects, reading and writing a sentence), and psychomotor ability (following a three-stage command and a drawing task). A score of below 24 is generally accepted as evidence of cognitive impairment. The AMT has 10 items and covers orientation, memory and attention, but does not assess language or psychomotor ability specifically.

Some people can score highly on the AMT or MMSE, but have difficulty with social activities and other aspects of daily life. They may be in the early stages of dementia; may be suffering from a frontal lobe pathology, or have some other organic problem. In such instances a short cognitive assessment will be inadequate. For example, Mrs Derbyshire in Case Study 4.1 scored poorly on the MMSE because it is a language-based test and she had a specific language problem, not because she was demented. Mr Singh (Case Study 4.2) scored poorly because his first language was not English, and depression may have been affecting his score. People with good verbal skills may score well on a screening test and 'hide' real difficulties with everyday memory (such as remembering appointments, shopping lists and conversations), which are due to dementia. More specialist assessments – which may take place in a memory clinic – are designed to address these issues.

> **Case Study 4.1 Mrs Derbyshire's MMSE**
>
> Mrs Derbyshire was an 82-year-old widow and a retired shop assistant. She was identified by her GP at her annual health check as possibly suffering from dementia. According to her family, she was having difficulty buying groceries at local shops – sometimes returning with the wrong item. She was also nervous about using the phone, and had difficulty finding words and making conversation. She scored 14 out of 30 on the MMSE – a low score. However, she could still look after herself. Her house was spotless and her garden well tended. She could make Sunday roast for eight people with no difficulty. A specialist assessment at a memory clinic identified no health problems and no difficulties with non-verbal memory, problem-solving or practical daily living skills. However, she had severe language problems. A CT scan confirmed a diagnosis of Primary Progressive Aphasia – a progressive language impairment. For several years, Mrs Derbyshire continued to live on her own. Specialist advice from a speech and language therapist working with a social worker enabled her family to encourage her to make the best of her non-verbal abilities and provide support with communication where she needed it.

Monitoring treatment

The introduction of new drugs for the treatment of Alzheimer's disease, together with interest in memory retraining and rehabilitation work has resulted in tests being repeated to see if there is any change in cognitive function over time. Most of the commonly used tests (MMSE, CAMCOG) do not have alternative versions of the memory and concentration questions, and are not good measures of change because the practice effect of repeating the same test over time can lead to improved performance. Some tests, such as ADAS (Rosen, 1984) and MEAMS (Golding, 1989), do have alternative versions and should be considered if the purpose is to monitor change in memory and cognition.

Memory and cognition are not the only abilities that can respond to drug, psychological or environmental interventions. Behaviour and mood changes may be more readily noticed by clients and carers. Some of the ADL and IADL scales referred to earlier can be used to monitor changes of mood, especially those that have been refined or developed for people with dementia, such as the Cornell Depression Scale, which is rated by an observer (Alexopoulos *et al*, 1988), and Pleasant Events Scale – AD (Teri & Logsdon, 1991). The 15-item Geriatric Depression Scale (GDS, Sheikh & Yesavage, 1986) has a 'yes/no' format, which is easily completed by people with mild dementia.

Case Study 4.2 Mr Singh's individual assessment

Mr Singh, a retired nurse aged 70, has had a number of mini strokes and has been diagnosed as having MID. Recently he appears to have taken a turn for the worse, avoiding friends and social activities and sometimes not dressing or eating much. His wife is in poor health and their two children live away from the area. His sister in India died recently. He scored poorly on the MMSE (15/30). He also scored 12/15 on the Geriatric Depression Scale, indicating a strong possibility of depression. The CPN was concerned that these tests might be biased, as Mr Singh's first language was not English, so an individual assessment was devised with the help of Mr Singh and his wife, using an IADL scale. After three months' treatment for his depression he was once again able to eat and dress and had begun to enjoy family events, although he avoided some occasions with more distant acquaintances as he became embarrassed when he could not remember their names and faces.

Assessing quality of life

Quality of life measures, such as the QOL-AD (Logsdon *et al*, 1999), or Dementia Care Mapping (DCM, Kitwood, 1997), are used to monitor the effects of therapy programmes and care environments on clients' wellbeing. These approaches have particular value among people whose verbal abilities or cognitive impairments make it difficult for them to express their needs. The QOL-AD is a short checklist of items for use with clients and carers. DCM involves systematic observation of clients' behaviour in a care setting (usually a hospital, residential home or day unit) every five minutes over a number of hours on different days. The frequency of certain behaviours and the quality of interactions between clients and staff are rated according to a detailed schedule. A 'map' of care can then be produced with an overall rating of care for an individual or for the care setting as a whole. Ratings of care can range from +5 for 'high quality interaction and evidence of a therapeutic bond' conducive to a state of 'wellbeing' to –5 for evidence of 'severe ill being'.

Assessing caregiver needs

Most behavioural and ADL measures are completed by carers and can help identify the burden on the caregiver. They have tended to focus on the impact of behavioural problems and symptoms associated with different stages of dementia identified by health professionals.

Nolan and Grant (1992) and Nolan, Keady and Grant (1995) have developed tools for evaluating carer satisfaction (Carers Assessment of Satisfaction Index, or CASI); ability to manage (CAMI), and perceptions of difficulty (CADI). While not specific to dementia, they can be used with caregivers of people with dementia. They go beyond an assessment of carer strain based on ADL scales. They suggest that carers should be viewed as experts. Programmes aimed at carers should try to develop their expertise by increasing their knowledge, identifying areas of satisfaction, and increasing predictability in the tasks of caring (for example, by knowing when help will be available).

Planning services

Some measures, such as the CAPE and BASOLL, are structured in such a way as to identify those people experiencing problems who are most likely to be cared for in particular settings – own home, residential home or hospital. The CAPE (Pattie & Gilleard, 1979) was developed at a time when Health and Social Services care predominated, and the categories may not apply so readily to the burgeoning private residential and nursing-home sector. The BASOLL (Brooker, 1997) has been found to be sensitive to those with particularly challenging behaviour, and distinguishes between users of day hospital, respite and continuing care services.

Case Study 4.3 describes how a service planned the objectives of assessment and then decided on the best tools to use in their setting.

Case Study 4.3 A community health team's assessment methods

A new community mental health team was concerned that, after initial diagnosis of dementia, they did not have a standard method of assessing and monitoring needs that could be used by health and social worker members of the team, and which included carer needs. The day hospital team for dementia assessment had been using the MMSE and MEAMS, but realised most people had been diagnosed by the community mental health team or memory clinic long before they got to the day hospital. The two teams wanted to work together on clarifying the purpose of their assessments and using appropriate tools that avoided duplication. They held an away day to discuss the aims of each team and select the most appropriate assessments.

The community mental health team continued to use dementia assessment and screening tools to help with referral to the memory clinic for diagnosis, and to train primary-care staff in their use. The day hospital would repeat the MMSE, but felt it should focus more on functional rehabilitation and on building self-esteem. The occupational therapists undertook to increase the home visits they did and started to use a process-orientated IADL assessment (the Kitchen Task Assessment) to develop rehabilitation and risk management approaches for people who had difficulty cooking. The nurses began to assess mood more systematically, using the Cornell Depression Scale when people started attending and as part of the evaluation of their therapy groups.

Both teams had a major role in supporting vulnerable carers and ran a number of psychoeducational groups for them. They decided to use the same carers' assessment to identify carers' needs and assess the effectiveness of these groups.

Issues to consider in choosing an assessment

Despite developments that have made cognitive and behavioural assessments more specific to particular needs, there are limits that need to be borne in mind when a choice of assessment is being made, whether for an individual client or as part of a service assessment, evaluation or research project.

Are you using the assessment for the purpose intended?

Most assessments cannot be used alone for diagnostic purposes. Some are screening tools indicating a need for more detailed assessment. Some ADL scales rate severity of a problem, but not why the problem has occurred. English-language-based assessments may discriminate against people from ethnic minority groups and people with poor reading skills, so ADL or IADL assessments may be more useful. Some ADL and behaviour-rating scales may be biased in terms of gender, social class or culture. For example, a kitchen task may be meaningless for someone who has never cooked in their life, and measures that give high scores to 'independence' will make it hard to assess someone who believes increased dependence on their family is an appropriate late-life adjustment. It is important for users of an assessment to know for what purpose and for which people it is designed, and to be honest about this with clients.

If an assessment is being carried out as part of a diagnosis, rather than as a baseline for treatment, what does the service do with the information, and how does it share it with the person assessed?

Can the assessment be used as a basis for care-planning and treatment?

Cognitive and behavioural assessments have been used most often for diagnostic and service-planning purposes. They identify impairments and may highlight strengths and weaknesses. Health- and social-care staff need to be confident in using and interpreting the assessments they use; understand how to use them as a basis for setting goals and planning care, and be able to share this with clients and their carers.

Can the assessment be used with people from minority ethnic groups?

Some tests have been validated for use with certain communities (Rait *et al*, 2000a; 2000b). Certain behavioural, ADL and carer measures may not be culturally relevant. Clarity about the purpose of particular assessments; sharing ideas about useful measures, and using individualised goal-planning approaches (see Goudie, 1990) with people from the communities using the service are essential elements of tailoring dementia services to meet diverse needs.

Can the assessment be used with younger people with dementia?

Most of the existing screening tools and dementia-specific cognitive and behavioural assessments have been designed for older people. However, there are around 17,000 people under 65 years with dementia in the UK. Rarer dementias seem to be more common in younger people, therefore cognitive assessment and diagnosis of dementia usually involves longer batteries of tests and more neurological investigations. The use of behavioural and ADL measures for care planning or rehabilitation are likely to be inappropriate in terms of age and interest. Assessments will need to focus on occupational and child-care abilities. There may be overlap in assessment and treatment issues between teams.

Other issues to consider include pre-diagnostic counselling; test circumstances, and how feedback will be given. For more detail on this see Lamers (Chapter 5, Memory Clinics).

Summary

Cognitive and behavioural assessment may be key elements in assessment of and screening for dementia. Developments in assessment mean that there is now a wider range of specialist tools that can be used in a more holistic way to assess not only cognition and behaviour, but also mood, quality of life and carer satisfaction. Health and social care staff need to think carefully about where and how best to use these tools so that they are useful not only for diagnostic purposes, but also for planning and evaluating treatment, and for monitoring change and the quality of care environments.

References

Alexopoulos GS, Abrams RC, Young RC & Shamoian CA, 1988, 'Cornell Scale for Depression in Dementia', *Biological Psychiatry* 23, pp271–4.

Baum C & Edwards DF, 1993, 'Cognitive performance in senile dementia of the Alzheimer's type: The Kitchen Task Assessment', *American Journal of Occupational Therapy* 47, pp431–8.

Brooker D, 1997, *BASOLL – Behavioural Assessment Scale of Later Life*, Speechmark Publishing/Winslow Press, Bicester.

Bucks RS, Ashworth DA, Wilcock GK & Siegfried KS, 1996, 'Assessment of activities of daily living in dementia: Development of the Bristol Activities of Daily Living Scale', *Age and Ageing* 25, pp113–20.

Carswell A, Dulberg C, Carson, L & Zgola J, 1995, 'The Functional Performance Measure for persons with Alzheimer disease: Reliability and validity', *Canadian Journal of Occupational Therapy* 62, pp62–9.

Folstein MF, Folstein SE & McHugh PR, 1975, 'Mini-mental State Examination. A practical method for grading the cognitive status of patients for the clinician', *Journal of Psychiatric Research* 12, pp189–98.

Golding E, 1989, *Middlesex Elderly Assessment of Mental State,* Thames Valley Test Company, Tichfield.

Goudie F, 1990, 'Goal Planning: Towards Meeting Individual Needs', Stokes G & Goudie F (eds), *Working with Dementia*, Speechmark Publishing/Winslow Press, Bicester, pp91–8.

Hodkinson HM, 1972, 'Evaluation of a mental test score for assessment of mental impairment in the elderly', *Age and Ageing* 1, pp233–8.

Hope RA & Fairburn CG, 1992, 'The Present Behavioural Examination (PBE): The Development of An Interview to Measure Current Behavioural Abnormalities', *Psychological Medicine* 22, pp223–30.

Kitwood T (ed), 1997, *Evaluating Dementia Care: The DCM Method*, 7th edn, Bradford Dementia Group, Bradford.

Lawton MP & Brody E, 1969, 'Assessment of older people: self-maintaining and instrumental activities of daily living', *Gerontologist* 9, pp179–86.

Logsdon R, Gibbons LE, McMurry SM & Teri L, 1999, 'Quality of Life in Alzheimer's disease: Patient and caregiver reports', *Journal of Mental Health and Ageing* 5, pp21–32.

Nolan MR & Grant G, 1992, *Regular Respite: an Evaluation of a Hospital Rota Bed Scheme for Elderly People,* Age Concern, London.

Nolan MR, Keady J & Grant G, 1995, 'CAMI: a Basis for Assessment and Support with Family Carers', *British Journal of Adult/Elderly Care Nursing* 1(3), pp822–6.

Patel V & Hope RA, 1992, 'A rating scale for aggressive behaviour in the elderly', *Psychological Medicine* 22, pp211–21.

Pattie AH & Gilleard CJ, 1979, *Manual for the Clifton Assessment Procedure for the Elderly (CAPE)*, Hodder & Stoughton Educational, Sevenoaks.

Rait G, Burns A, Baldwin R, Chew-Graham C, Morley M & St Leger S, 2000a, 'Validating Screening Instruments for Cognitive Impairment in Older South Asians in the UK', *International Journal of Geriatric Psychiatry* 15, pp54–62.

Rait G, Morley M, Burns A, Baldwin R, Chew-Graham C & St Leger S, 2000b, 'Screening for Dementia in Older African-Caribbeans', *Psychological Medicine* 30, pp957–63.

Rosen WG, Mohs RC & Davis KL, 1984, 'A new rating scale for Alzheimer's disease', *American Journal of Psychiatry* 141, pp1356–64.

Roth M, Tym E, Mountjoy CQ, Huppert FA, Hendrie H, Verma S & Goddard R, 1986, 'CAMDEX: A standardised instrument for the diagnosis of mental disorder in the elderly with special reference to the early detection of dementia', *British Journal of Psychiatry* 149, pp698–709.

Sahakian BJ, 1990, 'Computerised assessment of neuropsychological function in Alzheimer's disease and Parkinson's disease', *International Journal of Geriatric Psychiatry* 5, pp211–13.

Sheikh JI and Yesavage JA, 1986, 'Geriatric Depression Scale (GDS): recent evidence and development of a short version', Brink TL (ed), *Clinical Gerontology: A Guide to Assessment and Intervention*, pp 165–73, Haworth, New York.

Spiegel R, Brunner C, Ermini-Funfschilling D, Monsch A, Notter M, Puxty J & Tremmel L, 1991, 'A new behavioural assessment scale for geriatric out and inpatients: The NOSGER (Nurses' Observation Scale for Geriatric Patients)', *Journal of the American Geriatrics Society* 39, pp339–47.

Teri L & Logsdon R, 1992, 'Identifying pleasant activities for Alzheimer's disease patients: the Pleasant Event Schedule-AD', *Gerontologist* 31, pp413–16.

Terri L, Truax P & Logsdon R, 1992, 'Assessment of behavioural problems in dementia; the Revised Memory and Behaviour Problems Checklist', *Psychology of Ageing* 7, pp622–31.

CHAPTER 5

Memory Clinics

Carolien Lamers

A T THE STAGE WHEN MEMORY PROBLEMS, other cognitive deficits or personality changes become more noticeable, some clients and their carers will seek guidance as to the nature and origin of these problems from their general practitioner. GPs can find it difficult to diagnose the nature of the deficits, and might need to refer on to a more specialist service. Depending on the age, type, duration and severity of the problems, a GP has several options for onward referral. These include neurology, geriatric medicine, old-age psychiatry, clinical psychology, older adult community mental health teams or, in some places, memory clinics.

Memory clinics may also be known as dementia clinics or cognitive disorder clinics. 'Memory clinic' is considered a more acceptable name than 'dementia clinic' as the word 'dementia' still has a lot of stigma attached to it and some people might find it off-putting to attend for an assessment. Others also feel that terms like 'dementia' and 'cognitive disorder' reflect the loss-deficit model that prevails in the medical world. Memory clinics usually provide an assessment that reflects an holistic approach to the person, their social network and the disease.

What is a memory clinic?

There is a great variability in the 20 or more clinics across the UK as identified by Wright and Lindesay (1995). Some are based in primary care settings; others operate within mental health clinics or specialist hospital departments. The clinic may be a full-time service based in a specially allocated building, or only run at specific times with specialist practitioners who normally work in other settings.

Most memory clinics provide a multidisciplinary, out-patient, specialist service in diagnosing and early detection of neuro-degenerative disorders. Their remit may consist of assessment, follow-up, brief psychological, social and pharmaceutical interventions and longer-term support. The purpose of the clinics also depends on the way their funding has been arranged. The majority receive funding from within the Health Service, and focus mainly on providing a clinical service. Others receive money to carry out research or to undertake pharmaceutical trials.

Some clinics only see people from their local area, while others take referrals from a wider region. Referrals to the clinic may come direct from the GP or any other medical professional, or from members of the mental health teams. Waiting times can vary between six weeks and six months.

Who works in a memory clinic?

The specialist nature of the work carried out in a memory clinic is reflected in the multidisciplinary make-up of the team. Usually there is a medical person available: a neurologist, geriatrician, or consultant in old-age psychiatry. The other members of staff may be a clinical or neuropsychologist, speech and language therapist, occupational therapist, nurse or social worker. Sometimes a worker from the Alzheimer's Society is attached to a clinic and can provide further information and support. All of the staff will have an interest in organic brain disorders, and will have received some specialist training.

Who is seen in a memory clinic?

Each clinic will have their own criteria as to which referrals they will accept. Some operate an age limit; others will only accept referrals from other colleagues in the service after they have carried out the routine screening and there is still a diagnostic uncertainty. Some clinics accept self-referrals from people or carers who have anxieties about their brain functioning, although the GP will usually be informed about this.

What happens in a memory clinic?

Assessment at a memory clinic can take from one hour to a whole day. The person is invited to bring any aids they might need (such as glasses or hearing aids) and their current medication. A carer who knows them well; a partner, child or other relative or friend is welcome, as they can help clarify the presenting problems and address any other concerns.

Pre-diagnostic counselling

Being referred to a specialist service because someone is experiencing memory or other related problems can be an anxiety-provoking experience for both the person and the carer. Some people worry about suffering from a dementia syndrome or a brain tumour; others describe their experience as 'going mad'. They may subject themselves to lengthy and repeat assessments if they think successful treatment will result. It is unethical to exploit this, and important to be honest about the pros and cons of assessment. Not everyone with a diagnosis of dementia can be prescribed cognitive enhancers. There may be implications following a diagnosis for a person's work, driving and social activities.

It is important for the person to be given the opportunity to explore their feelings and thoughts, and to address any questions or queries they may have. This information is useful in the assessment process as it indicates the level of insight, but even more so in the discussion as to whether or not the person would like to be informed of the diagnosis, and whether the carers can be informed of the outcome of the assessment.

The person could be asked the following questions:

- How serious do you think the problem is?
- Do you know others with similar problems?
- Does a family member have a history of memory loss?
- How would you feel if you were found to be suffering from a degenerative condition?
- What is your greatest fear?

It may be relevant to ask the carer the same questions.

At this stage the person also has the opportunity to ask questions about the assessment process itself, as well as what happens if a diagnosis

Case Study 5.1 Mrs Hudson's dilemma

Mrs Hudson was not sure whether she wanted to know what was wrong with her. She was worried that she had the same illness as her mother, who became 'senile'. Her mother ended up being unhygienic in her self-care and had wandered the streets in her nightie. Mrs Hudson became upset recalling these events. The psychologist said she could appreciate why Mrs Hudson was not sure, and that thinking of her mother must be upsetting. However, care has improved over the years and, if she was found to be suffering from a similar illness to her mother's (and this was not proven yet), then there was no evidence to say that she would experience the same difficulties as her mother. What would not knowing mean to Mrs Hudson? She would wonder every day, every minute what lay ahead. What would it be like knowing and being able to prepare for the future?

of a dementia syndrome is reached. It might be necessary to point out the consequences of the assessment. For example, if a positive diagnosis is made and a person is still driving, the staff might advise the person to stop driving, and the relevant authorities will need to be informed. In cases where the client is still working, the employer might need to be told. In some rare cases, more likely early-onset dementia, where there might be a hereditary factor, insurance companies might want to be informed.

Based on this information, the person can refuse to continue with the assessment. This outcome could leave staff with some difficult ethical dilemmas, especially when a dementia syndrome is suspected and the person could endanger themselves and others.

Some people deny the existence of any problems and attribute their failing memory to an ageing process. This can make the assessment complicated as the person might be unwilling to accept the investigations. For many families this is a difficult time as they are worried about their relative, but cannot readily access services as the nature of the problems is unclear. In these instances, preparatory work is even more crucial in order to gain the confidence of the person. Sometimes a member of staff at the memory clinic – often the nurse – can go on home visits and thus develop a relationship that will enable the assessment process to be undertaken in the future.

It is true to say that pre-diagnostic counselling does not happen in each clinic. Some professionals might hold the view that these discussions cannot be held with people with a suspected dementia syndrome, as they will be unable to comprehend or recall the information (Drickamer & Lachs, 1992). Others fear that the topic can upset the person and might cause depressive feelings. Some professionals might make assumptions about the impact the condition has on the person's ability to make informed judgements, and could override the person's rights to confidentiality and inform the carers of the person's condition.

Others oppose these views and feel that the person has got an intrinsic right to be informed if they so wish. Not knowing what is wrong can lead to all sorts of unrealistic fantasies, and can be as upsetting as knowing. The client might have enough insight to understand the information, provided it is shared in a common language, avoiding jargon. They might also see the benefits of informing their relatives.

Assessment

The range of cognitive and behavioural assessments that may be carried out in a memory clinic was described in Chapter 4. These determine the presence and severity of impairments. Another aspect of the assessment is collecting information that helps in making a diagnosis. This information is required so that any other conditions that might imitate or aggravate a dementia syndrome can be eliminated.

The different specialists involved in the clinic usually carry out their own specific assessment.

Physical examination

In order to exclude any underlying physical causes of the cognitive deficits, a physical examination will be carried out by the doctor in the team. Depending on their specialism, the focus might vary somewhat, but a range of the basic bodily functions will be assessed. This is combined with a routine blood test, which will look for anaemia, thyroid dysfunction, presence of infections, diabetes and so on. Sometimes further tests might be requested, depending on the outcome of the initial physical investigations These could include certain types of brain scan (CT [computerised tomography] or MRI [nuclear magnetic resonance imaging] scans), or specialist medical assessments to exclude stroke or Parkinson's disease.

Any physical conditions that might aggravate the cognitive functioning will be treated. Reassessment at some point in the future might be undertaken to assess the extent to which the treatment of the concurrent condition has alleviated the cognitive problems. A diagnosis might be established at this point in time.

Collateral History

Most clinics will invite the person to bring along someone who knows them well. They will be asked about the history of the presenting problems as well as the extent of the difficulties. The extent to which the two stories overlap can in itself be a useful tool in the assessment process. The aspect of insight on the part of the person is thus assessed. Brief personal history, schooling and work history are also taken; the latter to get an idea of the level of functioning of the person before the problems became apparent. Also, different levels of functioning for somebody who left school at the age of 14 and a university lecturer would be expected.

Neuropsychological assessment

The previous level of functioning is also taken into consideration when the results of the neuropsychological assessments are interpreted. The neuropsychologist will ask the person a range of questions, and ask for certain tasks to be performed in order to assess the functions that can be affected by an organic brain syndrome – ie, memory, language, orientation, constructional tasks, abstract/reflective thinking and visuospatial abilities. More detailed neuropsychological assessment might be needed if the findings of the initial assessment are ambiguous. (See Chapter 9 for a description of neuropsychological impairments.)

Sufficient attention must be given to the factors that might affect performance. Has the assessment been set for a time and place which is as stress-free as possible? Can enough time be given so as not to rush the person? Does the assessment have to be given in one go, or can it be broken into shorter sessions to avoid fatigue? If it has to be completed in one day, can the person have a break for a drink or snack? Does the person have glasses or a hearing aid with them if they use them? What plans can be made for rescheduling an assessment if the person is physically unwell?

Language assessment

Language functioning can be assessed in more detail by the speech and language therapist, who will conduct a specific language assessment looking at the ability to express oneself, understand spoken and written language, reading and writing. (See Chapter 10 for more on the assessment of language and communication.)

Functional assessment

The effect of the cognitive deficits on the day-to-day functioning in terms of self-care and managing one's affairs can be assessed by an occupational therapist.

Mental health assessment

In order to exclude other psychiatric conditions that might induce or mimic a dementia syndrome, a mental health assessment is carried out. The person is asked about their mood, their thoughts and feelings. Low mood or depression can mimic a dementia syndrome, but can also co-exist, particularly if the person is aware of their failing abilities. Other specific psychiatric presentations, like delusions and hallucinations, are checked. The presence of the above does not exclude a diagnosis of a dementia syndrome, but can help in the diagnostic process to define the type of illness the person suffers from. As some of these symptoms can be distressing it is important to treat them too.

Carer's assessment

The impact of the cognitive deficits on the support system must also be taken into consideration. Caring for a person with even the mildest dementia syndrome can be stressful for any carer, be they a spouse, child, other relative or friend. Each category of carer may experience particular difficulties. The nature of the pre-existing relationship can be important in this.

All the information collected is not only useful for diagnostic purposes, but can also be of help when considing different kinds of interventions and support.

Case Study 5.2 Mrs Hudson's assessment

Mrs Hudson had agreed to attend two assessment sessions and also had an MRI scan at the local hospital. She was physically fit for her age apart from hypertension, for which she received treatment. There were no abnormalities in her blood test. On the cognitive assessment it appeared that she was a bright woman, which fitted in with her career as a teacher and then headmistress. The memory assessment supported her subjective complaints of memory problems. The other findings indicated that she also had problems in abstract thinking and perception; however, her ability to understand spoken and written language and to express herself was still working to a satisfactory level. Her mood was low and she was obviously anxious about the assessment. This could have affected her performance, but would not account for the all deficits. The MRI showed global atrophy in keeping with age, and some vascular changes.

Sharing the diagnosis

Based on all the information gathered above it might be possible for the memory clinic team to reach a diagnosis. Some clinics operate rigid criteria based on internationally agreed guidelines (such as DSM 4-R or ICD10).

Any treatable conditions that might interfere with the cognitive function will be treated first before a final diagnosis is made. Not all clinicians communicate the diagnosis to their clients. Sometimes the referring agent is informed of the outcome of the assessment process and it is up to this person to convey the information to the person. Some studies (Rice & Warner, 1994) have shown that it depends on the level of dementia as to whether or not the person is informed. People with more advanced dementias are less likely to be informed. This practice might reflect a general belief about the nature of the condition, as described above.

In clinics where the diagnosis is shared with the person, a special meeting will be arranged, and depending on the findings from the pre-diagnostic counselling, the wish of the person to be informed or not will be taken into consideration. In sharing the diagnosis it is important for the clinic staff to avoid jargon; to take the process step by step, and to ensure that the person has the opportunity to ask questions. Often a follow-up appointment with one member of the team in the person's home setting will be offered to ensure that the information shared is understood. Many people find a letter describing their assessment and the results very helpful. Writing reports for colleagues in user-friendly language can reduce the need for two separate reports.

Case Study 5.3 Mrs Hudson's diagnosis

Mrs Hudson met with the psychiatrist and psychologist to discuss the findings. They began by explaining that she was physically fit and that they had not found a treatable condition that could account for the problems she was experiencing. She was a bright woman and was still competent in many areas. There were, however, memory problems and difficulties in logical thinking and problem-solving. She also might experience trouble in recognising objects if they were presented from an unusual angle. This all indicated that there were several areas in the brain affected, and this could not be seen as a sign of normal ageing. Her history of high blood pressure and the findings on the scan began to point at a problem with the blood circulation in her brain. All the findings pointed to a dementia syndrome of possible vascular nature. This meant that her condition would get worse over time, but she was likely to have periods of stability.

Post-diagnostic counselling

The post-diagnostic counselling begins at the time the diagnosis is shared with the person and can be seen as a psychological intervention in itself. The way this is done is important and can set the scene for the counselling that might be needed afterwards. Not all clinics provide this service themselves, but any professional involved in the care of the person with the established dementia can undertake this. It is important to go over the information that has been shared and to clarify any areas where there is doubt. The person might need reminding about the information. The memory problems and the higher cortical functions may complicate this process. Although in principle counselling techniques can be applied, the tempo of the counselling and speed of processing needs to be adapted. The links need to be made more explicit and step by step. Written or pictorial information can be helpful.

Questions about the future can be expected as well. Will my memory get worse? Will I start to wander? Will I become aggressive? Do I need to go into care? The area of prognosis needs to be dealt with in an honest manner, yet there must be careful consideration of the impact this may have on the needs of the person and their carers.

Case Study 5.4 Mrs Hudson discusses the findings

The nurse went to visit Mrs Hudson to discuss the findings. Mrs Hudson was upset at the thought that things would become worse, but was also reassured that she might function at the same level for some time. She still thought about her mother, but felt that she was better off knowing than worrying all the time. She had started to discuss power of attorney with her children and was planning a visit to her brother in Australia together with her sister. The nurse discussed possible practical ways to aid her memory and to begin consolidating routines to ensure she could stay at home for as long as possible. Other practical help could be organised when the time arose. Mrs Hudson wanted to meet other people in a similar position and the nurse said she would find out what was available. The nurse felt that her low mood at the time of the assessment was a normal coping response and not indicative of a depressive episode.

Genetic counselling

Genetic factors are involved in only certain types of dementia syndromes – for example, Huntingdon's disease or a familial type of Alzheimer's disease, usually early-onset. If relatives want to find out whether or not they carry the gene, they can be referred on to the appropriate services where they will receive genetic counselling.

Support and therapy groups

Some post-diagnostic counselling can be done in groups with people suffering from a similar condition. People generally find it very helpful to meet others specifically to discuss their situation. They can share the experience itself; how they feel, and what sort of emotions accompany the illness. The impact the condition may have on their lives and on the lives of their relatives will be relevant areas to share.

Intervention

The range of interventions possibly available through a memory clinic is discussed in the next chapters.

References

Drickamer MA & Lachs MS, 1992, 'Should patients with Alzheimer's disease be told their diagnosis?', *New England Journal of Medicine* 326, pp947–51.

Rice K & Warner N, 1994, 'Breaking the bad news: what do psychiatrists tell patients about their illness?', *International Journal of Geriatric Psychiatry* 9, pp467–71.

Wright N & Lindesay J, 1995, 'A survey of memory clinics in the British Isles', *International Journal of Geriatric Psychiatry* 10, pp379–85.

Further reading

Wilcock G, Bucks RS & Rockwood K (eds), 1999, *Diagnosis and Management of Dementia: A Manual for Memory Clinic Teams*, Oxford University Press, Oxford.

CHAPTER 6

A Person-Centred Understanding

Graham Stokes

U NTIL NOW OUR JOURNEY OF DISCOVERY has rightly focused upon the assessment of cognitive and functional abilities and the identification of pathology. In other words, we have considered the evidence for a diagnosis of dementia. We now progress our understanding by moving on from 'pathology' to 'person', for our reasoning cannot be limited to 'they've got dementia'. The explanation for behaviour and emotions in dementia is far more complex.

The medical disease model of dementia

The biomedical model assumes a causal relationship between brain disease and dementia, yet this fails to acknowledge the complexity of the human experience of dementia. Just because we possess indirect evidence of pathology in the brain, this is not sufficient explanation for the incompetence, emotions and challenging actions we encounter. The brain diseases described in Chapter 2 (The 'Dementias') devastate a person's cognitive world (for example, the domains of memory, intellect and language) and determine entry to a state of degrading incapacity. Move beyond the limits of the cognitive paradigm and psychological and environmental factors need to be considered when explaining the rich tapestry of behaviour observed in dementia. For too long the assessment and care of people with dementia has been dominated by the despair and negativity that seeps from a disease model that views the deteriorating profile of behaviour solely in terms of progressive neurological destruction. This has produced a culture of care that is little more than 'warehousing' – namely meeting the basic physical needs of a person and making them as comfortable as possible (Sixsmith *et al*, 1993).

Why the biomedical model continues to hold sway cannot be ascribed to a single explanation. A complex interaction of factors serves to weave a fabric that successfully clothes what Kitwood (1989) called the 'standard paradigm' with credibility and authority which, at best, it only partially deserves. It starts with our personal dread of dementia. We need to know that it will be somebody else who will end their days roaming around a building lost and bewildered, experiencing the degradation of being soiled, not even knowing their own children. To know it will not be us, we invoke the 'social distance'. This is the distance we place between ourselves and any group of people who threaten or frighten us. As a result we never get to know them, yet the distance between us is fertile ground for the growth of myths and stereotypes – beliefs we know to be true because we never seek evidence to the contrary. Hence we *know* that those who dement must always have been odd, quirky or eccentric; lived unhealthy lifestyles; watched an excessive amount of television (Highfield, 2001); inhabited a world of dark secrets, or maybe they were always muddled and scatterbrained. As we are 'as pure as the driven snow' and so competent in all we do, we know we will never dement. The social distance works to our advantage, but it detaches us from those with dementia. We see them not only as being unlike ourselves in their current state, but we regard them as never having been truly like us.

The process of detachment has commenced – a process that is perpetuated during the course of care – for where is the encouragement to cross the social distance, not to find out what a person was once like, but to determine what they are currently experiencing in the midst of their dementia? A number of factors conspire to corrupt our understanding of a person with dementia, and act as a significant impediment to crossing the distance. In turn the dominance of the medical model is secured (Table 6.1).

Yet the person does remain. The medical model cannot explain all. The person may become increasingly difficult to see, and their behaviour

Table 6.1 *The impediments to crossing the social distance that promote the dominance of the biomedical model*

- The identification of neurological diseases to 'explain' dementia, along with sophisticated methods of radiological investigations, has encouraged a biotechnical understanding of dementia and confirmed the authority of medicine.

- The medical model talks only of disease and symptoms. The 'person' is squeezed out of existence, so everything a person does after the diagnosis of dementia is attributed to the diagnosis. This is so easy to understand that we find its simplicity seductive (ie, 'A' causes 'B').

- The more we see people as different from ourselves, the more we believe their behaviour is the product of disease.

- The words of troubled and distressed families can so often reinforce the belief that we are concerned solely with the signs of pathology. We hear of 'shells', 'shadows' and 'bodies'. A person once known and loved, now departed. As such they acquire the status of a non-person.

- Cognitive destruction profoundly limits communication, and this serves to impede the search for understanding beyond the reporting of symptoms.

- A neurological framework encourages a comforting 'no-blame' culture of care. Whatever a person with dementia does (or does not do), we can absolve ourselves of any responsibility by blaming the disease.

may bewilder and exasperate us, but they are 'people of full human worth and value, despite their disability' (Woods, 2000).

Person first, dementia second

People are a rich tapestry of needs and preferences, hurts and fears, doubts and insecurities, strengths and weaknesses, likes and dislikes, emotions and habits. 'Unfortunately, this inner world is often denied to people with dementia' (Stokes, 1995). Yes, with the passage of time, their unique individuality will be distorted, disfigured and will ultimately disappear. However, as many have observed, people with dementia retain for so long 'the basic core characteristics that made them the person they always were' (Bell & McGregor, 1995). As we endeavour to appreciate the personalities and life histories that individuals bring to their dementia, we cannot allow the destruction of language, memory and reasoning to be an insurmountable barrier to understanding who people with dementia are and why they do what they do. If we make contact with the person behind the barrier – a barrier constructed by neurological disease and reinforced by the complicating effects of ill-health, medication and disability (Figure 6.1) – we are offered the opportunity to 'stand the prevailing opinion of dementia on its head and assert that much behaviour in dementia is not meaningless, but meaningful' (Stokes, 1995).

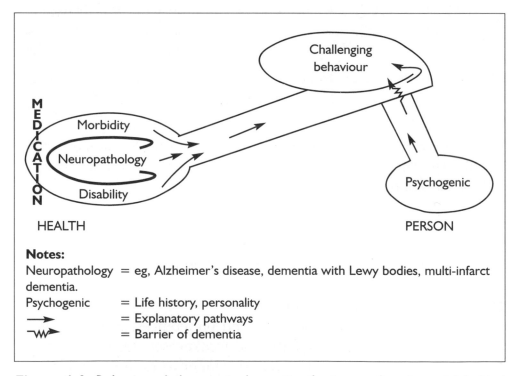

Figure 6.1 *Behavioural changes in dementia: the person (psychogenic) behind the barrier of cerebral disease (neuropathology)*

The person centred model of dementia

What is meant by the term 'a person with dementia'? It can often appear to be little more than a glib statement. At other times, reference to a person with dementia appears to be a contradiction in terms. Families protest that they do not recognise and cannot relate to what they see before them. 'Each time I came home, she was less and less like my mother' – the words of a loving daughter, *Daily Telegraph*, 1 April 1998. 'For all the intimate familiarity of that face and body ... I did not feel his presence beside me, only his absence' (Morris, 1995).

Yet it is not the person who is lost, but the relationship as once known, which is no more. The person, despite their multiple cognitive disabilities, remains an 'active agent', interpreting their experiences, addressing their needs and expressing how they feel. How we framework a person with dementia is shown in Figure 6.2.

---

1   We accept a person who is unique (eg, having a life history, fears, joys and habits).

2   We acknowledge a person with whom we share much in common.

3   We recognise the subjective experience of dementia – a world of not knowing.

Figure 6.2 *The person-centred model of dementia*

1 True to myself, getting on with life

We acknowledge the uniqueness of the person – a person who, despite their dementia, will live their life as they see fit, addressing their habits and doing their best. As such, perplexing actions can be the consequence of a 'comfortable behaviour' or a motivational response that is appropriate to the present, but has been distorted by the limits of their neuropathology.

'Comfortable behaviour' is the way we are. A challenging continuation of who we have always been. It is our automatic ways, topics of conversations and daily habits. To partake in them feels right. If you enjoy your own company first thing in the morning; need time to gather your thoughts; never wish to have people around – how well would you cope in the social world of care? Could this be why a person with dementia walks away or resists efforts to get them to sit down with others? Do you eat everything placed before you? There are personal anxieties. Some people sleep with a light on, a door open; others would never venture into a lift. To what extent do we know those with dementia?

Maybe the actions are evidence of motivational responses to resolve perceived practical problems, or to be effective in daily life. There are stories of people cutting the grass with scissors or 'mowing' the lawn with a vacuum cleaner. Many practitioners know of clients who have placed electric kettles or plastic bowls instead of saucepans on their cookers. Case Study 6.1 illustrates well-intentioned motivation.

Case Study 6.1 Harry's probable Alzheimer's disease

'H' had slashed the new sports jacket his wife had purchased only the day before with a pair of scissors. Her interpretation was that, in retaliation for removing his favourite, albeit soiled, suit he had been deliberately malicious and destructive.

'H' could never settle. He would roam around the house taking little time to rest. As a result his wife would leave sandwiches in the kitchen so he could 'graze' while walking. During the course of eating, 'H' had more than likely inadvertently squeezed the contents of a sandwich down the front of his jacket, and then lacked the intellectual capacity to successfully effect his desired course of action. He could not tell his wife of his accident, because of significant speech impairment. Nor did his reasoning decrements enable him to sponge the stain. Instead he had picked up a pair of scissors and cut out the piece of cloth. A man with no regard for his clothing, or a person who remained concerned about his appearance?

---

2 A common bond

We acknowledge a unique individual, yet this is founded on a basic premise – a fundamental that asserts that, as we are, a person with dementia remains a feeling, sentient being with whom we share more in common than that which separates us. What distinguishes us is our contrasting intellectual powers. What we share are those essential needs that define our humanity: the essence of what it means to be human. These include not only physiological needs, but also fundamental psychological needs, such as security, self-regard, sociability, curiosity and activity – needs that are observed to motivate behaviour during our earliest formative years.

A state of agency remains. This does not mean, however, that actions can be predicted or readily associated with the inner world of motivation. For example, the experience of low-grade chronic pain in dementia and the need to be pain-free may present as shrieks and shouts; irritability; spiteful actions; calling out for a parent; withdrawal, or apparently aimless walking. Insecurity may result in calling out, searching or questioning. As was noted long ago by Hebb (1955), needs are 'an engine but not a steering wheel'. We do not see easily recognisable motivational behaviour. Instead we observe behavioural ruin and chaos. The result is a dysfunctional and, at times, grotesque distortion of goal-directed communication and conduct.

The person presents as altered, but personality at its most fundamental level has not changed. Yes, prevailing actions are at variance with the person once known. But these actions are an inadequate measure of the essential core of the person. An unadventurous, somewhat timid, woman lived a sheltered life. Within the undemanding limits she set for herself she was safe and content. Untroubled, she was a gentle, pleasant woman, always willing to help others. Tragically, she shows signs of early dementia. She finds herself in an assessment unit. A strange, noisy, invasive environment. Unsurprisingly, her need to be secure drives her to leave the unit. When prevented from doing so she becomes violent. She spits at staff blocking her way. Actions inconsistent with her pre-morbid self? Behaviour 180 degrees away from the gentle woman she used to be? Yes. But a person lost? No. She would always have acted in this manner if her need for security had been violated. It is just that having constructed a life that was without threat, she was never driven to acts of desperate self-protection. Her need for security led her to adopt a sheltered lifestyle; now it has resulted in violent acts of self-destruction.

A person with dementia may not only act out their needs. Alternatively, they may attempt to communicate, unfortunately with little success. We hear their words, but are we listening? They may ask for their parents. Miesen (1993) developed the hypothesis that Alzheimer's disease generates 'strangeness', which in turn activates attachment behaviour that manifests as 'parent fixation' – an expression of need that cannot be automatically dismissed as evidence of confusion, confabulation or delusion. Instead it can be seen as the communication of the need to be in the proximity of another person who provides tenderness and a sense of safety and security. As we know, parents provide without question care and love and, during troubled times, they are a comforting source of protection. As people with dementia live with a 'kind of psychological pain whose persistence and intensity we can scarcely envisage' (Kitwood, 1989), they may reach out for such compassion and utter the words, 'Where's my mother'. For example, Bayley (1998) wrote of a trip with his wife, Iris Murdoch, 'The drive to London was a nightmare. Iris protested wildly. We were going the wrong way – she must get out – where was her mother? Screams and tears.'

Asking to go home may represent an attempt to communicate a need to belong or be safe; a woman who asks for her children may be desperately communicating a need to be needed. Demanding to go to work could be a plea to be useful and occupied. Asking for a husband or wife suggests a need for emotional warmth, companionship or sexual intimacy. Concealed messages abound. Goudie and Stokes (1989) introduced resolution therapy as a way of gaining access to this world of need and feeling.

Understanding increases the prospect of solution. Yet even when resolution is not possible, as the behaviour loses its mystery it can generate tolerance. Actions remain challenging, but others can now appreciate that they are not living with, or caring for a 'shell' of what went before.

3 A time of not knowing

This person whom we now know – unique, but with whom we share so much – experiences a subjective reality that is difficult for us to comprehend, for to dement is to enter a time of 'perpetual not knowing'. A state of rarely, if ever, knowing where you are, how you arrived, who others are and, possibly of greatest significance, what will happen next. This is disorientation. Faced with an inability to store information and learn, the unfamiliar never loses its mystery. A pervasive sense of uncertainty prevails. And this state is often experienced in a world that is unsupportive and depersonalised (Kitwood, 1990). It may be endured while living alone or in the company of people with dementia – not *other* people with dementia, for a person with severe dementia does not appreciate they are dementing.

Instead, their social world is an aggregation of others who are unlike them – people who act in unpredictable, asocial and intimidating ways. Any one of them may act out, but in the absence of a capacity to retain novel information, they will forget within moments their own errors and misdemeanours.

A tragedy for people with dementia is that, even when they remain in the place that is most familiar to them – namely their own home – surrounded by people who know them best – their family and friends – as time passes and memory disintegrates according to the principle of Ribot's Law (that which is experienced last, is lost first), any vestige of security is destroyed. The familiar becomes unfamiliar; frighteningly and increasingly so. Partners and children are no longer recognised, a home ceases to be reassuring. Strangeness now prevails.

For some, the subjective experience of dementia is to occupy both a world of knowing and not knowing. The neuropathological destruction of most recent memories leaves only those from the past, and it is these that constitute the foundation of a life to be lived again. Once more they will have parents, young children and jobs to go to. It is not that they bring their past into the present, the past is all there is. Yet where are these loved ones? Why are they not where they should be? Curiosity, if not torment, generates a determination to search. We see confusion; they experience frustration and yearning. A time passed, but again restored to the 'here and now'. It is not that they experience a chronologically determined unfolding of historical events, re-experiencing their lives as lived. Instead, their acting out of personal history encompasses overlearned ways of being and themes (such as parenthood, work, home, parents and partners) of emotional significance. Memories that become fixed, 'secured' and, in dementia, constitute a world not of belief, but of entrenched and enduring conviction. A reality very different from our own – one that may possess little internal logic – but which is, nevertheless, a reality as meaningful to them as ours is to us.

Why most enter a state of uncomplicated not knowing, while others relive their past with unfailing conviction is not known. Stokes (2000) believes the explanation is not neuropathological, but is likely to be psychological, residing in the 'need to know' of those whose pre-morbid personality was 'controlling'. A person who was ill at ease and insecure when 'not knowing' would rather 'do it themselves' than rely on others – a way of being founded on a mistrust of others and a tendency to 'fear the worst'. In order to remove uncertainty and ward off dangers, control was secured through the pursuit of knowledge. In dementia, however, recent memories and knowledge are eroded. All a person possesses to understand their world is information which, from our perspective, is from years long past. As they trawl their minds in an effort 'to know' – at times in response to 'private events'; on other occasions in response to external cues (for example, a dementing woman sees her mirror image as 'mother', which in turn prompts confused 'searching') – their 'time distant' memories become a 'restored reality' (Sherman, 2001). We struggle with their confusion. They experience loss and bewilderment.

Conclusion

This is the subjective life of a person with dementia. Cheston and Bender (1999) argue for a model of dementia that addresses the subjective state of experience and feeling. This chapter represents an attempt to comprehend this internal world. We acknowledge an individual who makes decisions and initiates actions, while residing in a reality that resonates 'not knowing'. A person who may be sorely misunderstood. As they live their lives, express their needs, address their problems, it is we who also become exasperated and bemused.

References

Bayley J, 1998, *Iris*, Gerald Duckworth, London

Bell J & McGregor I, 1995, 'A Challenge to Stage Theories of Dementia', in Kitwood T & Benson S (eds), *The New Culture of Dementia Care*, Hawker Publications, London.

Cheston R & Bender M, 1999, *Understanding Dementia*, Jessica Kingsley, London.

Goudie F & Stokes G, 1989, 'Understanding Confusion', *Nursing Times* 85(39), pp35–7

Hebb DO, 1955, 'Drives and the CNS (Conceptual Nervous System)', *Psychology Review* 26, pp243–54.

Highfield R, 2001, 'Watching television linked to Alzheimer's', *Daily Telegraph*, 6 March.

Kitwood T, 1989, 'Brain, Mind and Dementia: With Particular Reference to Alzheimer's Disease', *Ageing and Society* 9, pp1–15.

Kitwood T, 1990 'The Dialectics of Dementia: With Particular Reference to Alzheimer's Disease', *Ageing and Society* 10, pp177–96.

Miesen BML, 1993, 'Alzheimer's Disease. The Phenomenon of Parent Fixation and Bowlby's Attachment Theory', *International Journal of Geriatric Psychiatry* 8, pp147–53.

Morris E, 1995, 'The Living Hand', *The New Yorker,* 16 January, pp 66–9.

Sherman M, 2001, personal communication.

Sixsmith A, Stillwell J & Copeland J, 1993, 'Rementia: Challenging The Limits of Dementia Care', *International Journal of Geriatric Psychiatry* 8, pp993–1000.

Stokes G, 1995, 'Incontinent or Not? Don't Label: Describe And Assess', *Journal of Dementia Care* 3(1), pp20–21.

Stokes G, 2000, *Challenging Behaviour in Dementia*, Speechmark Publishing/Winslow Press, Bicester.

Woods RT, 2000, 'Foreword: Person-centred Care – Success Stories?', in Benson S (ed), *Person-Centred Care,* Hawker Publications, London.

CHAPTER 7

The Environmental Setting of Dementia

Graham Stokes

NEUROPATHOLOGY IS INEXTRICABLY woven into the patterns of an individual's life history and personality, and suffered as a subjective experience. The person remains an active agent initiating, yet also *responding,* to events. While they determine much from within, they are also affected by their life setting. Their environments may serve to exaggerate, even create, dysfunctional behaviours. Hence, when understanding dementia, environmental circumstances and the quality of social relationships are essential components of the explanatory 'equation'.

What is the environment?

When we consider the environment, we do not confine ourselves to the buildings within which people live ('the built environment'); we also address what is of even greater significance when understanding behaviour in dementia – namely the world of attitudes and interpersonal relationships ('the social environment'). We also distinguish between the 'situation' and 'context'. The 'situation' is the face-to-face contact between those who live with or care for a person with dementia that occurs within a specific location. The 'context' is the environmental setting within which these people live and work. In professional care we make reference to custom and practice, rules and regulations, and the quality and availability of material and human resources. With family care, contextual factors pertain to such issues as marital history and family dynamics. For example, a loveless marriage is not transformed into a tender, tolerant relationship simply because one of the partners develops dementia.

Contextual features may be of great significance. These may create the circumstances responsible for situational triggers, and in turn may obstruct desired remedial intervention. Looking beyond a limited view of the environment so as to take into account contextual influences is known as 'behavioural ecology'.

The built environment

The built environment refers to the material world, yet the contribution architectural design might positively make to the lives of people with dementia is not at all clear (Keen, 1989). While Marshall (1998) confidently asserts 'that the built environment can have a fundamental effect on a person with dementia ... design for people with dementia has not been subjected to the scrutiny of research in the same way as medication, for example'.

The contribution of building design

Despite the paucity of research, the basic position of all workers is that buildings in some way influence the behaviour of people who live within them, even though opinion remains largely intuitive. Lawton and Simon (1968) put forward the 'environmental docility' hypothesis. In other words, the more incompetent and vulnerable a person is, the more their behaviour is controlled by the environment that surrounds them.

The implications of this line of argument for those with dementia is clear. They are among the least competent people. If they find themselves in unsupportive surroundings, a marked proportion of their dependent and dysfunctional behaviour can be attributed to their environment. Many years ago, Lindsley (1964) proposed the prosthetic environment, wherein skills and abilities that are damaged or lost are compensated for by the provision of environmental prostheses. 'If behaviour is deficient, the environment could be altered in order to produce effective behaviour.'

In similar vein, the potential value of the 'empathic model' of design has been explored by Pastalan (1984). The model's general principles attempt to create living arrangements that are enabling rather than disabling:

1 'Organised space as stimulus'. If recognition, recall or understanding have deteriorated, make a design message available through more than one sensory modality. An example is a dining room, where the clatter of knives and forks, smell of food and sight of crockery, dining tables and chairs all declare, 'this is where you eat!'.
2 'Organised spaces as orientation'. Any space should have a singular and unambiguous use, for people with dementia are less able to resolve ambiguities.

Misidentifications and mistaken beliefs can be resolved if care practice and settings present the person with clear and unambiguous messages. Stokes (2000) describes how a creative intervention that employed the principles of the 'empathic model' of design resolved the violent reactions of a woman with severe dementia whose childhood had been marked by abuse.

Other design features that contribute towards quality care and enable relative well-being, yet if absent may either cause or contribute to the onset of challenging behaviour and exacerbate dependency, include:

• *The intimacy gradient.* In a residential or nursing home people need a gradient of settings that have different degrees of intimacy. A bedroom is most intimate; a lounge in a group-living unit less so; a communal sitting-room more public still; the front entrance area most public of all. All buildings that accommodate people need a definite gradient from 'front' to 'back', from the most public spaces at the front to the most intimate areas at the rear.

Without a gradient of intimacy, care actions are often inappropriate to context. Intimate behaviours such as toileting may take place next to a front entrance, while access to a sleeping area may be open to visitors and staff on arrival. Shared bedrooms result in people waking up with a stranger in their midst. Such a poor fit between a person and their environment can result in distressed, defensive and uncooperative behaviours, for the subjective experience is both perplexing and intimidating.

- *Corridors.* The time a resident spends between rooms can be as important as the moments spent within rooms. A corridor that is long, devoid of natural light and bare of furnishings is consistent with our worst ideas of what is meant by 'institution'. Spivack (1967) described how long corridors distort the perception of distance; interfere with verbal communication; obscure perception of the human figure and face, and generate anxiety and fear as a result of feeling enclosed. The potential for disorientation, conflict and unsafe interaction is described by Pennington (1996). To design out these effects, corridors should be kept short; they should benefit from natural light, and be areas of interest. Themed corridors, 'full of things to look at and touch' (Bignall, 1996), encourage people to linger with purpose. Such corridors cease to be experienced as passages and become very much a part of the living space of the building, supporting the rhythm of daily life.

- *Interior design.* Condemning people with dementia to live in anonymous, sterile surroundings compounds their inability to transform the unfamiliar to the familiar, and hence ensures the strangeness of their existence. While orientation cues (such as colours, symbols, sounds and aromas) may only benefit the minority, there is nothing to be lost, and possibly something to be gained, by building directional prosthetics into interior design. If just one person is spared the indignity of roaming around wet and soiled then such intervention is to be valued.

- *Decision points.* Distance and complexity contribute to problems of disorientation, wandering and toileting difficulty. Netten (1989) found, unsurprisingly, that the more light there is, the more able a resident will be to find their way around. Meaningful landmarks also aid orientation. Unhelpful designs are when there are a lot of 'meaningless decisions', such as when there are long corridors with lots of doors, or when several short corridors create a 'maze' effect.

The building: an obstacle or opportunity?

While buildings clearly matter, it is naïve to propose a deterministic view of the relationship between buildings and people who live in them. Such crude architectural determinism is flawed, for buildings and designs are only as important as the manner in which they may or may not be used, and the constraints and opportunities they present. Buildings can hinder or help the provision of quality care: in extreme cases they can prevent it but, to state the obvious, buildings by themselves cannot provide it (Pennington, 1996). Arie (1987) asserts that 'given a basic adequacy of material environment', quality of care depends on staff morale, motivation and training. Hence it can be confidently argued that the quality of the interpersonal environment is of greater importance than the physical, for negative staff attitudes will negate the effects of even the best architectural design (Woods, 1996). Conversely, institutionalisation is as much, if not more, the consequence of staff attitudes and actions as it is the result of architecture.

The social environment

There is clear convergence between the various accounts that address the positive characteristics of caregiving (see Table 7.1), yet the poor quality of life for elderly people with dementia in permanent care has been demonstrated time and time again. Devaluation, invalidation and dehumanisation have often been described (Woods, 1995).

Lindesay *et al* (1991) make reference to a process of 'institutional maintenance' whereby procedures and routines benefit the smooth-running of the institution rather than the needs of those who live in them. Kitwood (1990) refers to the 'processes and interactions that tend to depersonalise a sufferer from dementia' as the malignant social psychology – a significant non-biological influence on dementia that is founded on the biomedical

Table 7.1 *Positive characteristics of care*

Care is concerned primarily with the maintenance and enhancement of personhood. Providing a safe environment, meeting basic needs and giving physical care are all essential, but only part of the care of the whole person. (Kitwood, 1995)	1 It values the person with dementia as a full human being. 2 The individualisation of care requires getting to know the whole person. 3 It achieves effective two-way communication. (Woods, 1995)

framework of a person suffering from a brain disease for which nothing can be done. Therapeutic nihilism dominates as carers believe the person does not experience life or suffering and requires only basic physical care.

The malignant social psychology
In 1990, Kitwood proposed these two fundamental equations:

SD = NI + MSP   (Senile Dementia is compounded from the effects of Neurological Impairment and of Malignant Social Psychology)

$(NI)_a \leftarrow$ MSP   (Neurological Impairment in an elderly person attracts to itself a Malignant Social Psychology)

In so doing he articulated what was known intuitively – namely that when 'we follow any person's dementing illness carefully, observing its course in the realities of everyday life, it is extremely difficult to conclude that we are simply witnessing the inexorable consequences of a process of degeneration in nervous tissue' (Kitwood, 1996). However, in other writings, Kitwood (1993) acknowledged a complex interaction between five factors that had been previously elucidated by Stokes and Allen (1990):

Dementia = Personality (P) + Biography (B) + Neurological Impairment (NI) + Health (H) + Social Psychology (SP).

It is Kitwood's contention that the progression of dementia depends primarily on the interplay between neurological impairment and the person's social world.

While Kitwood's concept of malignant social psychology is most applicable to the inadequacy of care, it needs to be acknowledged that malignancy is to be found in the social grouping of dementia. In other words, anyone who has dementia may be distressed or devalued by the actions of those with whom they live alongside, as well as by those who care for them.

Abuse, maltreatment and insensitivity – a continuum of malignancy
Much has been said about the insensitive and dehumanising 'taken for granted world of care', that is driven by good intentions, yet unwittingly corrosive – a malignant social environment eloquently described by Tom

Kitwood and his colleagues at the Bradford Dementia Group. Yet not all care that is destructive and damaging is without malevolent intent. While levels of elder abuse (for example, neglect, physical assault, sexual abuse and financial exploitation) are thankfully low – or at least the reporting of episodes is uncommon – abuse of older adults is 'acknowledged as a social problem in need of remediation' (Kingston & Reay, 1996).

Between the extremes of obvious abuse and the taken-for-granted world of malign care, Stokes (2000) describes maltreatment – deliberate, knowing actions that are damaging to those who are vulnerable. What distinguishes these from abusive acts is that abuse, when exposed, is condemned, while maltreatment is condoned and accepted. To the enlightened, the cases described by Stokes (ibid) resonate with a sense of abuse, not impoverished care. Yet the actions of tying people down, communal toileting and 'bathing batches' were known, tolerated and advocated by the involved caregivers, sometimes for years.

Wellbeing in dementia

We do not need to be told when the quality of dementia care is poor, where people are treated en bloc, as if they have the same needs; where little effort is made to preserve dignity; where they are 'treated as a passive, inanimate object to be cleaned and changed in a dehumanising manner' (Woods, 1996), for those with dementia are superb barometers of the quality of care. Kitwood (1995) describes the 'sense of deadness, apathy, boredom, gloom and fear; most of those being cared for appear to have given up hope; their last resort being an occasional moan, or shout, or angry outburst.'

Where negative emotion dominates we talk of a state of ill-being (Buckland, 1997) – a state characterised by a desire to leave, restless agitation, screaming, anger and overt hostility. However, what is often observed is a state of apparent indifference, not overt distress or hostility. Is it true, then, that those with dementia are unaffected by their experience? Many people have commented on how struck they are by the emotional indifference of those with dementia (eg, Gilleard, 1984), the interpretation being that these people are untroubled by the experience – evidence that when insight is lost the 'worst is behind them'. Yet how wrong we have been. Their apparent indifference is consistent with what is known of victim responses. Victims of abuse, regardless of its nature, rarely, if ever, fight back. In the beginning there may have been resistance and protest, but eventually this is replaced by passive resignation. They are weak, the abuser is powerful. They no longer resist or recoil, but enter a world of semi-depressed withdrawal, seemingly indifferent to their fate.

It is to be hoped that people with dementia are not victims of abuse, yet they are victims of circumstances. They do not wish to be among those who, in their eyes, are not like them, or to be deprived of personal respect. They do not wish to be alone in a mysterious world of not knowing. While in the beginning they may have protested – hitting out, shouting, trying to leave – they soon present as accepting and indifferent. Yet this cannot be interpreted as evidence of positive adjustment and defined as 'settling down'. We should be as concerned for those who are passive, silent and disengaged as we are for those who are demonstrably suffering.

A culture of care that frees itself from the shackles of the 'standard paradigm' and strives to maintain a state of relative wellbeing (Kitwood *et al*, 1995) is concerned with the quality of human relationships. It is culture founded not on principles of control, containment and management, but on sensitivity, empathy and resolution.

Yet the delivery of person-centred care is not easy. It is demanding and requires a greater degree of empathy and identification with the person with dementia than traditionally observed. That resident who is uncooperative, always resisting when we wish to take her to the toilet or to the dining table – is her behaviour that surprising? Does she deserve to be labelled as resistive? Would you willingly go with strangers, even if they smiled and tempted you with fine words? Behind the barrier of shattered memory and devastated understanding, that is who we are: strangers with little to offer other than mysterious intent. We protest they are people like ourselves, then expect them to do what we could never do. Not simply to go with those whom they do not know, but often to receive intimate care when they are incapable of knowing their own deficiencies. Not able to know because so much of our core self-care knowledge, such as bladder control and appropriate toilet use, is pre-memorial. In other words, the knowledge became part of our 'personal truth' before our earliest memories were laid down and hence can never be erased.

Similarly, what is it like to be stopped from leaving a building when all around is chaos and noise? Or finding someone in your home who reassures you that you are safe and then requests you sit down as you have nowhere to go. Despite the role and title of home care worker, this person will be perceived as a stranger. What would you have done if, on waking this morning, a person you had never seen before had told you to stay indoors? Might you have protested, attempted to 'escape', demanded to know their identity and that they should leave? You do not have to be dementing to act in such a way, but to do so when you are will result in others degrading your actions to the status of symptoms and labelling you as a 'changed person' – aggressive, violent, abusive, noisy and a wanderer.

An holistic model of explanation

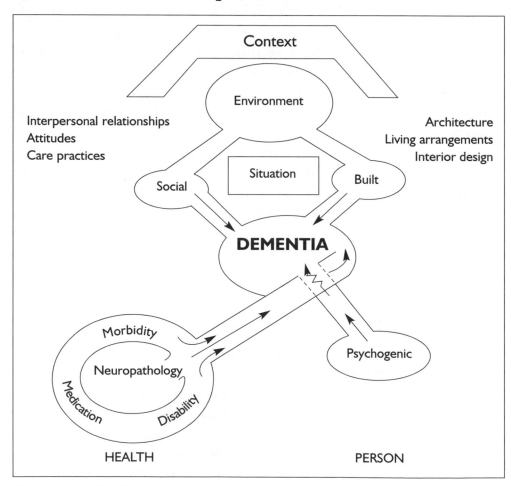

Figure 7.1 *The holistic person-centred model of dementia*

The model of understanding is complete – an understanding that is far removed from the reductionist explanation provided by the 'standard paradigm'. The explanatory pathways responsible for what we know as dementia are clear to see in Figure 7.1.

We have moved far away from a nihilistic disease model to the description of a framework that helps us to develop cultures of care that acknowledge the person and identify the potential for change. The pathways enable us to reveal the struggles of those who are attempting to live their lives in the face of neurological adversity in settings ill-equipped to either respect their personhood or respond to their needs. No explanation of dementia can stand without reference to these roots.

References

Arie T, 1987, 'Personal Communication', in Norman A (ed), *Severe Dementia: The Provision of Longstay Care*, Centre of Policy on Ageing, London.

Bignall A, 1996, 'Look and Learn: Designs on the Care Environment', *Journal of Dementia Care* 4, pp12–13.

Buckland S, 1997, 'How Well is Well-Being in Dementia?', *PSIGE Newsletter* 60, pp8–10.

Gilleard CJ, 1984, *Living with Dementia*, Croom Helm, London.

Keen J, 1989, 'Interiors: Architecture in the Lives of People with Dementia', *International Journal of Geriatric Psychiatry* 4, pp 255–72.

Kingston P & Reay A, 1996, 'Elder Abuse and Neglect', in Woods RT (ed), *Handbook of the Clinical Psychology of Ageing*, John Wiley, Chichester.

Kitwood T, 1990, 'The Dialectics of Dementia: With Particular Reference to Alzheimer's Disease', *Ageing and Society* 10, pp177–96.

Kitwood T, 1993, 'Person and Process in Dementia', *International Journal of Geriatric Psychiatry* 9, pp541–5.

Kitwood T, 1995, 'Cultures of Care: Tradition and Change', Kitwood T & Benson S (eds), *The New Culture of Dementia Care*, Hawker Publications, London.

Kitwood T, 1996, 'A Dialectical Framework for Dementia', in Woods RT (ed), *Handbook of the Clinical Psychology of Ageing*, John Wiley, Chichester.

Kitwood T, Buckland S & Petre T, 1995, *Brighter Futures*, Anchor Housing Association, Kidlington.

Lawton MP & Simon B, 1968, 'The Ecology of Social Relationships in Housing for the Elderly', *Gerontologist* 8, pp108–15.

Lindesay J, Briggs K, Lawes M, MacDonald A & Herzberg J, 1991, 'The Domus Philosophy: A Comparative Evaluation of a New Approach to Residential Care for the Demented Elderly', *International Journal of Geriatric Psychiatry* 6, pp727–36.

Lindsley OR, 1964, 'Geriatric Behavioural Prosthetics', in Kastenbaum R (ed), *New Thoughts on Old Age,* Springer, New York.

Marshall M, 1998, 'Therapeutic buildings for people with dementia', in Judd S, Marshall M & Phippen P (eds), *Design for Dementia,* Hawker Publications, London.

Netten A, 1989, 'The Effect of Design of Residential Homes in Creating Dependency Among Confused Elderly Residents', *International Journal of Geriatric Psychiatry* 4, pp 143–53.

Pastalan L, 1984, 'Architectural Research and Life-Space Changes', in Snyder K (ed), *Architectural Research,* Van Nostrand Reinhold, New York.

Pennington R, 1996, 'Blowing the Whistle on Bad Design', *Journal of Dementia Care* 3, pp24–6.

Spivack M, 1967, 'Sensory Distortion in Tunnels and Corridors', *Hospital and Community Psychiatry* 18.

Stokes G, 2000, *Challenging Behaviour in Dementia,* Speechmark Publishing/Winslow Press, Bicester.

Stokes G & Allen B, 1990, 'Seeking an Explanation', Stokes G & Goudie F (eds), *Working with Dementia,* Speechmark Publishing/Winslow Press, Bicester.

Woods RT, 1995, 'The Beginnings of a New Culture in Care', Kitwood T & Benson S (eds), *The New Culture of Dementia Care,* Hawker Publications, London.

Woods RT, 1996, 'Institutional Care', in Woods RT (ed), *Handbook of the Clinical Psychology of Ageing,* John Wiley, Chichester.

CHAPTER 8

Behavioural, Ecobehavioural and Functional Analysis

Graham Stokes

HAVING ESTABLISHED THE COMPLEX ORIGINS of behaviour, systematic and *direct* observation may be very useful in successfully identifying reasons for the appearance and maintenance of a person's disruptive conduct. The objective is to establish whether there is a relationship between the behaviour and its setting.

Several methods have been used to observe behaviour, all of which are 'time expensive' for they require professional carers to dedicate time to the exercise of reliable observation and recording. Despite this very real limitation, the rich potential of behavioural analysis has been acknowledged by several specialists in dementia care (eg, Stokes, 1990; Perrin, 1996).

Behavioural analysis is often referred to as an ABC analysis:

A = Activating event or situation (the technical term is Antecedents)
B = Behaviour
C = Consequences

We want to know when the behaviour occurred, where it took place, what was happening at the time, and what was the response of others? We are attempting to determine whether the behaviour is triggered by events or being maintained by the consequences of behaving that way. However, from what we know of dementia, storage deficits invariably militate against the maintenance of behaviour by a learned appreciation of the consequences that will follow, at least in cases of advanced dementia.

Behavioural analysis is, however, no longer a crude, mechanistic study of the environmental controls of behaviour. As we shall see, it places the person at the centre of our understanding, yet accepts that, as the normal avenues of communication have been denied, we must probe deeper in order to uncover the person and their motivations.

The process of behaviour analysis

Target behaviour
The first objective is to determine which behaviour is going to be the focus of analysis. It is advisable to choose a single behaviour in order that a thorough understanding of this 'target' behaviour is achieved in terms of its environmental setting and the meaning it may possess for the person.

Another reason for selecting a single behaviour is that successful resolution may exercise a positive effect above and beyond the targeted intervention in terms of both the person's wellbeing and the responsiveness of the social environment to their wider needs.

Consideration should also be given as to whether the most troublesome behaviour should be the initial target for analysis and potential intervention. To show staff that needs can be met and as a result behaviour changes, it may be wise to choose a relatively 'easy' target. An apparently minor success can motivate carers and foster a climate of positive expectation.

Behavioural description
It is important to provide an accurate definition of the target behaviour to be observed and recorded, thereby avoiding 'fuzzy', vague statements. To keep personal opinion and interpretation to a minimum it is best to describe the behaviour in precise detail – a process known as 'pinpointing' (Stokes, 2000). Everybody involved with the person then knows exactly what they are having to monitor, because the definition so carefully detailed is *agreed* by all.

Recording methodology

The ABCs are recorded each time an incident is observed although, as Perrin (1996) notes, it is only in an ideal world that we can observe and record a behaviour throughout the day or night. Instead, we may employ momentary time sampling where a person's behaviour is observed at predetermined points of time. Alternatively, the nature of the behaviour may dictate that we select a specified period each day – say an afternoon or an hour each morning – and record each episode within that time-frame. Whatever method is selected, and obviously the greater the length of time or number of observation points, the more accurate the picture revealed. It is essential that:

- All staff are aware that the behaviour is being monitored.
- All information is recorded as near to the time of the incident as possible, as it is easy to forget the exact circumstances if recording is left until later.

The collection of information on possible contributory factors can be displayed on a record chart similar to that below.

Day, Date & Time	Duration	A	B	C	Background

The information on day and time may reveal a temporal pattern (for example, 'sundowning', see p158). For certain behaviours it is not frequency, but duration, which is of most significance, for example:

- The duration of an episode of noise-making
- The length of time of agitated pacing.

The A (activating) column records what was happening immediately before the target behaviour was observed. What had the person been doing? What was happening in the surrounding environment at the time? Who was present?

If we are confronted with noise-making we would need to record:

- The whereabouts of the person under observation
- A description of the surroundings
- What had been happening prior to the incident?
- Who was around at this time?
- Who was *not* around at this time?
- How did the person appear?

In the B (behaviour) column we do not simply tick or state 'yes' to demonstrate that the behaviour occurred. Instead we describe precisely what happened:

- Did the person seem aware of their actions?
- Did they appear agitated, distressed or indifferent towards their own behaviour?
- Was the noise-making intelligible or not?
- Did they appear to be communicating?

The C (consequences) column details what occurs immediately after the incident:

- What was the response of others to the person's behaviour?
- What was said to the person?
- What was the person's reaction to the attention of others?

The background column covers circumstantial details that enable us to place the immediacy of the ABCs into a broader situational and contextual framework. For example, has anything happened during the day (or night) that may have caused upset? Has there been a recent change in routine, or the introduction of medication? Has the person recently moved to new surroundings? Is there somebody absent who is typically present? Has there been a recent change in environmental conditions (eg, temperature or interior design)?

If background information is not collected then essential reasons for why B may be occurring, as well as why the person was in situation A, and why they and others reacted at C in the manner they did, will be missed. When we address the broader setting within which behaviour occurs, we are moving into the realm of behavioural ecology. To meet a person's needs it may be that a fundamental restructuring of the overall environment is required. The need to look beyond a limited view of the environment is revealed by the plight of Jack (Case Study 8.1).

An ecobehavioural analysis (Emerson, 1993) provides an accurate and detailed description in terms of how often the behaviour occurred;

Case Study 8.1 Jack's Plight

Jack was often found wet in the corridors of the residential home (B). Although this could happen throughout the day, it was most frequently observed around mid-morning. Behavioural analysis recorded that, prior to wetting himself, he would be walking around the building agitated and apparently confused (A). He would be demanding to go home and protesting 'I am fed up with this place, this isn't my home.' His confusion was either ignored or corrected by staff who were busying themselves with household tasks (background). On discovering him wet, staff would at last devote time to him. There was now a task to be done. They would take him to the bathroom to be washed, and then to his bedroom to be changed (C) – actions that Jack often resisted.

When it was suggested to staff that they were ignoring Jack's needs, and that his agitated 'confused' behaviour was in fact the actions of a man desperate to communicate his need for the toilet ('I am fed up with this place, this isn't my home. The toilet should be there and it's not, I NEED THE TOILET!'), they readily understood. They appreciated that they needed to give him more time; pace their communication; listen to the messages, but the home manager wished all the beds to be made, the residents' rooms to be tidied and the dining tables wiped down before the mid-morning drinks were served at 11.15 am (the behavioural context). Only physical care tasks could be accommodated within this schedule. Any suggestion that flowed from the behavioural analysis would inevitably flounder on the bedrock of institutional inflexibility, unless the analysis also included an appreciation of the behavioural ecology and in turn recommended contextual changes.

the circumstances in which it arose; the consequences for the person, and any relevant contextual features.

The procedure

The observation and recording of the target behaviours should take place over a period of one to two weeks; in order to avoid making decisions on the basis of short-term fluctuations in behaviour. In other words, monitoring for just a few days may result in staff having unwittingly chosen a couple of good days or a particularly bad patch, thereby giving rise to misleading conclusions. Taking time to assess helps avoid unjust labelling and rash decisions, actions that may not only be unhelpful but may lead to even greater challenges.

This stage of behavioural analysis is known as the *baseline period*. It helps not only to identify whether a consistent pattern exists, but also the *frequency* of the challenging behaviour: that is, how many times the target behaviour occurred during the baseline period. Sometimes, if the behaviour is observed to have a low frequency, this provides evidence that carers have lost perspective (unless the challenge is the duration of the activity – for example, noise-making or pacing). Being confronted by a demanding, invasive behaviour can sap energy, erode tolerance and, as a result, appear unremitting. When the low frequency is discussed with the staff team, they may conclude that the behaviour is not a significant challenge warranting special attention. We continue to consider which needs are unmet at a time of dysfunctional conduct, but such understanding does not require the introduction of extraordinary arrangements.

If a genuine challenge exists, the frequency observed forms the baseline against which future change is measured. Whatever form intervention may take, the frequency of the target behaviour continues to be recorded so that success can be confirmed or denied – success often being a meaningful reduction in frequency, not the ideal of zero frequency. If there are no positive developments, the formulation was wrong and the intervention requires re-examination. Thus, the continued use of frequency recording does away with subjective impressions of whether improvement has occurred or not.

For a detailed and honest account of behavioural analysis see Perrin (1996).

Functional analysis

While the collection of ABCs provides us with a detailed description of the relationship between environmental events and behaviour, we cannot restrict ourselves to such a limited methodology. We must continue to frame our understanding in accord with the person and their needs. Yes, a behaviour occurs in a particular setting and it may be inextricably related to that situation and its broader context but, as we have already seen, actions are a function of the person and their motivations. Functional analysis builds on the empirical rigour of a behaviour analysis and addresses the purpose served by the behaviour.

Given our understanding of the person-centred model of dementia, it is unsurprising that researchers have identified 'the functional significance of even the most bizarre and serious behaviours' (Samson & McDonnell, 1990). Functional analysis does not restrict itself to an appreciation of the immediate antecedents and/or consequences of a behaviour, but attempts to gain an understanding of the meaning and, possibly, usefulness (ie, the function) 'of a particular behaviour, in a particular set of circumstances, for a particular individual' (Samson & McDonnell, 1990). As a result, the pursuit of explanations includes not only that which is observed but, following a detailed investigation of 'person variables', a functional analysis also addresses the importance of what are known as 'unobservables' (for example, life history, abilities, needs, feelings, individual characteristics, neuropsychological impairment, ill health and sensory losses). In other words, reference is made to the health and psychogenic pathways (Figure 6.1). Let us consider the trials of Mr Bryan (Case Study 8.2).

Case Study 8.2 Mr Bryan – a gentleman no longer

Mr Bryan had always been a reserved man. Not a person you could easily warm to. Stern, critical but, nevertheless, a gentleman. Always respectful and courteous. Once a successful businessman, he started to show signs of dementia in his late fifties. After a few years his wife was no longer able to cope with his deteriorated state and he entered a nursing home.

Mr Bryan would spend his days pacing the corridors. Agitated, he would engage with no-one. If approached he would stare and walk away. On many occasions he would try in vain to open the French windows that opened on to the garden. Often he would bang on the glass in frustration. One day, for his own safety, a nurse led him away and sat him by the television (A). Within moments he had walked over to a hazard cone placed next to the lounge door by a cleaner. Picking it up, he clubbed a frail dementing woman who was sleeping in a chair (B). He was immediately taken into the office (C), and the doctor was called.

The 'unobservables'

Mr Bryan had coped with dementia by avoiding others. He would isolate himself in his garden and work there for hours without a break. He would say that 'out there', pointing to his garden, 'I don't fail'. That was not actually so, but his errors and misjudgements were not readily apparent to him.

His wife described him as having always been arrogant, a man who had never suffered fools gladly and could not tolerate weakness in himself. It was these characteristics that underpinned the actions that broke his wife's tolerance. He would never write down messages; instead he would try unsuccessfully to remember them. He objected to the prosthetics introduced by his wife to help him locate household items and he would never use his daily diary of 'things to do'. His fear of failure and his need to be right always were also the reasons for his avoidance of others. He disliked the presence of his wife, for she would tell him of his mistakes. He avoided company, for he would forget names, fail to recognise people he should know, lose the thread of conversations and, most distressing of all, he would repeat himself. Caught in the crossfire of words, he would walk out. People were averse to him, not because he was shy, but because he had insight into what were for him intolerable failings.

As the years passed his wife became increasingly isolated. Her husband's conduct led others to feel awkward and ill at ease. Friends no longer visited, neighbours rarely called round. She felt abandoned. Unsurprisingly, Mr Bryan's avoidant, self-centred, yet progressively dependent, behaviour exceeded her capacity to care. Somewhat prematurely he entered a nursing home. Mr Bryan had responded to his failing powers by withdrawing from social contact. Ironically, he now found himself having to endure the presence of people every waking moment (context). It did not matter that there was little conversation to avoid, or that the absence of insight meant that his failings were now no longer acknowledged. He simply found people intimidating. He was driven to leave their presence. That fateful day, when his frustration knew no bound, he struck out.

A meaningless act and the outcome of disease, or a motivated act resonating meaning and function that was consistent with the man once known by all?

The use of 'unobservables' is essential for achieving an imaginative person-centred explanation and increasing the explanatory power of a functional analysis. This is a considerable advance on the radical behaviour perspective that tries to establish relationships between observable features of the person's environment, and then attempts to modify behaviour by changing that environment – an approach that is in essence inimical to person-centred dementia care.

Samson and McDonnell (1990) describe how functional analysis works in practice:

1 Conduct a detailed analysis of a person, their history and needs. Involve all who know them. Collect information on remaining strengths, as these may be the foundations for future change. Identify factors that predispose a person to act the way they do, as well as those environmental features that finally trigger the behaviour.
2 Form hypotheses about why someone is behaving the way they are.
3 Draw up a formulation from the competing hypotheses that represents your 'best guess'. This may contain one, or a combination, of the original hypotheses. Having decided upon the possible function of the behaviour, the formulation should also state how the present situation might be changed.

Within the framework of single case experimental studies, Moniz-Cook and her colleagues (2000; in press) demonstrate the value of functional analysis in helping to resolve toilet refusal, noise-making, agitation and aggressive behaviour.

Conclusion

Functional analysis must be founded on accurate observation and considered information-gathering, otherwise it is little more than 'armchair theorising'. As a result, seeking an explanation can be a lengthy process. Unfortunately, time is not always on our side and human resources do not always allow for a rigorous period of monitoring. It is also the case that 'silent' behaviours – for example, incontinence – and those that are 'continuous' as distinct from discrete – for example, confusion, nocturnal wandering and apathy-withdrawal – do not easily lend themselves to an ABC analysis. Yet we do not discard the methodology outright, for the approach imposes a structure on our thinking. It enables us to understand what may be triggering and maintaining a person's behaviour, as well as guiding us to the role of the broader context and the significance of the behaviour for the person.

Functional analysis is without a doubt a formidable weapon to be employed in the pursuit of positive person-centred work. The conceptual and methodological expansion observed in its development provides an effective counter to the criticisms that behavioural analysis is an inadequate approach to understanding a person with dementia.

References

Emerson E, 1993, 'Challenging Behaviours and Severe Learning Disabilities: Recent Developments in Behavioural Analysis and Intervention', *Behavioural and Cognitive Psychotherapy* 21, pp171–98.

Moniz-Cook ED, Stokes G & Agar S, in press, 'Difficult Behaviour and Dementia In Nursing Homes: Five Cases of Psychosocial Intervention', *International Journal of Clinical Psychology and Psychotherapy*.

Moniz-Cook ED, Woods RT & Richards K, 2000, Functional Analysis of Challenging Behaviour in Dementia: The Role of Superstition', *International Journal of Geriatric Psychiatry,* pp1–12.

Perrin T, 1996, *Problem Behaviour and the Care of Elderly People*, Speechmark Publishing/Winslow Press, Bicester.

Samson DM & McDonnell AA, 1990, 'Functional Analysis and Challenging Behaviours', *Behavioural Psychotherapy* 18, pp259–72.

Stokes G, 1990, 'Behavioural Analysis', in Stokes G & Goudie F (eds), *Working with Dementia,* Speechmark Publishing/Winslow Press, Bicester.

Stokes G, 2000, *Challenging Behaviour in Dementia*, Speechmark Publishing/Winslow Press, Bicester.

PART 3

RELEARNING AND REHABILITATION

CHAPTER 9

Neuropsychological Impairments and Rehabilitation Approaches

Una Holden & Graham Stokes

THE PURPOSE OF THIS CHAPTER is to challenge the despair associated with dementia – a condition that means inevitable decline and degeneration. Unfortunately, such pessimism is characterised by therapeutic nihilism, wherein rehabilitation is seen as an objective incompatible with the nature of the problem. However, if we establish the specific reasons why a person is dependent we learn that even profound cognitive changes may be helped by positive care actions.

Memory impairment

A cardinal feature of dementia is a profound storage deficit. Often referred to as short-term memory loss, it results in disorientation, repetitive questioning and poor task performance. An accepted therapeutic response when faced with a person who cannot remember is reality orientation (RO).

There can be few people working in dementia care who have not come across RO. Its origins can be traced to the work of James Folsom at a Veteran's Administration Hospital in the late 1950s (Taulbee & Folsom, 1966; Folsom, 1968).

Growth in the use of RO throughout the 1960s and 1970s (not only with people with dementia, but also with those suffering from mental illness and the affects of institutionalisation) led Hussian (1981) to consider RO to be the major psychological intervention employed in dementia care in the USA. A similar expansion in the use of RO occurred in the UK between 1975 and the early 1980s. However, 'interest began to wane as it all too quickly became clear that here was no miracle cure …' (Woods, 1994). This led to practitioners querying whether RO had a place in contemporary dementia care.

A decade ago, Holden (1990) argued that 'In the 1990s RO will be a 24-hour approach … minimising excess disabilities and promoting independent action.' In pursuit of these goals caregivers present accurate and detailed information in everyday conversation and provide a commentary on what is happening as they engage with the person.

Orienting people to their environment, both social and built, is a valued exercise. However, as carers find the repetitious presentation of information tedious and tiring, common sense dictates the need to use environmental cues (for example, pathfinder arrows, colours and symbols), as well as verbal orientation to assist performance and way finding. The challenge in all instances is that clients do not remember. They do not retain what they are told, nor can they remember the purpose of the environmental designs. A cue to assist recall is useless unless the person learns the association between the cue and the information it is supposed to convey. Without learning, the cue has no meaning: a red door is just a red door. Though some people eventually learn the cue/information association (see Bird *et al*, 1995) most do not. Hence the results of RO in counteracting the more disabling consequences of disorientation have been generally disappointing (Bleathman & Morton, 1994).

This has led professional caregivers to become cynical and to apply the techniques of RO in a rote, uninspired manner (Morton & Bleathman, 1988; Dietch *et al*, 1989). They also question why they are doing it anyhow, for 'RO doesn't work'. Yet what would be the measure that affirmed 'RO does work'? It cannot be the retention of information, for as a result of pervasive and profound memory impairment, it does not matter how often a person is told, they will never remember.

RO is a prosthetic therapy. It cannot resolve the underlying inability to learn. Instead it compensates for memory function that has been damaged. We support way-finding around the home by prompts and reminders; we regularly inform the residents of our and others' identities; we keep them in touch with the task at hand, and we let them know what is happening around them. They may not learn, but they are still able to achieve the valued goal of 'assisted independence' through the creation of this prosthetic environment.

Yet ideas move on. As we enter the new millennium a response to RO is that it is seen by some 'as a dehumanising behaviour modification technique, solely preoccupied with targeting symptom management' (Bleathman & Morton, 1994), and thus as fitting ill in the new culture of dementia care.

Those with dementia are lost and bewildered, we are not. We know they are safe and well; they feel only the unknown. It is the purpose of RO to provide reassurance to those who are suffering the distress of disorientation. We are there to salve troubled emotions and calm their anxieties by replacing 'not knowing' with awareness. Even if we do not observe demonstrable improvement in daily living performance, the knowledge that we have identified with their subjective pain and for valued moments promoted wellbeing means RO is worth practising. The person who is frightened by the strangeness before them does not wish to hear how enjoyable the day will be. Their fear needs to be acknowledged; the accuracy of their observations affirmed. This is the domain of person-centred RO – addressing the subjective experience of dementia; informing and thereby emotionally supporting clients at times of distress. Yes, they will be back again, as troubled as before. But this is the nature of dementia.

Focal neuropsychological impairments

In the process of identifying the causes of behavioural and intellectual changes it is vital to ascertain if there are specific areas of brain damage or impairment. This requires awareness of neuropsychological features and the potential failure of care programmes if allowances are not made for these. For instance, to supply written instructions to a patient with alexia, or expecting a person with an apraxia to dress is a guarantee of failure.

Disturbances of communication, sometimes referred to as *aphasia* or dementia speech, is often the result of left-hemisphere pathology. It can present in a host of ways:

- Agraphia or dysgraphia (custom and practice has led to 'a' or 'dys' being used interchangeably, both meaning 'lost' or 'damaged' function) – a disturbance of the ability to write.
- Alexia – an impairment in the ability to read.
- Acalculia – a disorder involving numbers and arithmetic in general.
- Amusia – an inability to understand, recognise or interpret music.
- Dysarthria – imperfect articulation, with possible difficulties in respiration, phonation, resonance, volume, rate, intonation or rhythm.

When assessing speech it is important to appreciate at least two kinds of problem:

1 Those whose problem is speaking and word-finding (expressive deficits), though comprehension is preserved. A problem of word-finding is often referred to as anomia.
2 Those who can speak, but the person makes little sense and has little or no comprehension (receptive dysfunction).

The ways to help those with impairment of speech are described by Enderby in Chapter 10.

Apraxias are disorders of coordination that are not the result of physical or sensory deficits. The person appreciates what to do, but the moment their actions come under conscious control, they experience difficulties. Apraxias can take several forms:

- Ideomotor – a person cannot make a simple gesture or single action, such as picking up a cup of tea or responding to the request, 'open your mouth'.
- Ideational – though aware of what is required, a person cannot carry out a complex task requiring a series of movements. The person either 'grinds to a halt' or the sequence is disordered.
- Constructional – here a person has difficulty putting things together.
- Dressing – attempts to dress result in disorganised actions as the person fails to relate clothing appropriately to their body.

On all occasions, comprehension is preserved and actions can be performed automatically. When pushing and shouting are observed, these are often attempts to make the correct movements or to express frustration at their inability to do so.

Case Study 9.1 Mary's 'aggression'

Mary was regarded as aggressive and an attention-seeker. Staff had to help her dress and wash. They became annoyed when she screamed and pushed at them and the flannel, clothes or whatever else they were holding. When she was at the table her apparent refusal to eat was accompanied by shouts and screams, which disturbed everyone.

There is a simple means to help those who are apraxic – *avoid direct instructions and encourage automatic responding.* For example:

- If giving a person a cup of tea, say 'I hope you're thirsty'.
- When presenting them with their meal, say 'Your lunch smells delicious'.
- When wanting a person to get into bed, you can say 'You're looking tired.'

When working with specific deficits:

- Ideomotor and ideational apraxias may also be aided by the use of pictorial rather than verbal guidance.
- Constructional apraxia will also be helped by pictorial prompts and helping people to think a step at a time. When providing activity, straightforward construction games can be useful too – for example, collages and simple jigsaws.
- Dressing apraxia may need several approaches to meet individual need:
  - Use of colour – for example, red tab on right shoe, yellow tab on left; green label on back of dress.
  - Place clothes in correct order for dressing.
  - Offer verbal guidance by talking a person through each stage.

- Without saying anything, or by talking about something else, help the person get started.
- Mime the appropriate action.
- Demonstrate by putting on the item of clothing; then hand it to the person without offering any instructions.

Agnosias are disorders of recognition that result in an inability to identify an object. Usually only one sensory modality is involved, yet there is never a true sensory defect. In other words, a person may be unable to recognise an object by vision even though their eyesight is unimpaired. There are a number of different types of agnosia:

- Visual agnosia is the commonest form. The person fails to recognise what they see. It is as if they have never seen the object before and cannot establish the item's meaning.
- Variants of visual agnosia are prosopagnosia – a lack of facial recognition, so the person is unable to recognise their family, friends or possibly their own face – and simultanagnosia – an inability to see things as a whole.

Case Study 9.2 Larry's prosopagnosia

Larry, aged 64 years, suffered a stroke. He seemed to have made a remarkable recovery, but his family were distressed and puzzled as he did not recognise any of them by sight and was unable to identify anything he observed. His intellect and memory were impaired – the problem was prosopagnosia.

Case Study 9.3 Philip's simultanagnosia

Philip examined a picture in a book and was unable to give an appropriate description. It was a wedding, but he only saw a woman's face and he was unable to shift his gaze or to take in the whole scene. The cause was simultanagnosia.

- Auditory agnosia is rare. The person believes that everyone is talking gibberish. Sounds can be equally meaningless.
- Tactile or astereognosis is a lack of recognition by feel alone.
- Spatial agnosia is an inability to find one's way around. A person may become lost when out or even within their own home.

Rehabilitation suggestions involve taking advantage of the unaffected senses:

- Touch is important with visual agnosia. Friends and family need to speak, use familiar perfume and encourage the use of logic to find the meaning of items.
- Auditory agnosia responds well to a slower delivery of speech.
- Spatial agnosia may be helped by drawing a plan of the home and asking the person to describe the décor and furniture in each room. Later they can be asked, 'What colour is the carpet in the bedroom?'; 'What are the curtains like in the lounge?'. The person may draw a house plan or map of their neighbourhood themselves. Within a care home, the colour-coding and theming of corridors can aid way-finding, as can the use of background music and aromas. The identification of a person's own room will be aided by the use of memorabilia and photographs unique to that person.

One-sided neglect presents in several different ways:

- Unilateral spatial neglect results in a person failing to see, feel or hear anything to one side. For example, they may not see the food on one side of the plate.
- Sensory inattention is when a person is unaware of stimuli applied to the neglected side of the body.
- Anosognosia is denial of disability, or denial of the damaged side of the body.

Recent work on neglect (Robertson *et al*, 1993; 1995) has identified ways that we might work with Jack (Case Study 9.4). He needs to be encouraged to place his right arm to the left side of any activity and to

Case Study 9.4 Jack's anosognosia

Jack was a difficult man to understand. He refused to use his right arm, would only partially dress and was always climbing into bed with someone else. He was generally very unpopular, even with his relatives. Jack would often complain that others were hitting him. He only appreciated the world to his left side, so his bed on the right did not exist, but the bed to his left did. He refused to admit that his disabled right arm was his. If it touched his body he would think it belonged to someone else and make accusations of assault. When his one-sided neglect was appreciated it was easy to understand why he would even refuse to dress the right side of his body.

visually locate it. Asking him to switch off a buzzer placed to the damaged side of an activity using his right hand (which can be moved across by his left hand) is another means of minimising one-sided neglect.

Frontal lobe syndrome arises when there is damage to the forebrain of the cerebral cortex. Though frontal lobe disorders differ from person to person, several neuropsychological changes are likely to occur, all of which add up to a disturbance of executive functioning:

- Perseveration – repetition of words, phrases, writing or actions.
- 'Stuck needle' syndrome – unable to shift 'set' and move on to other themes or activities.
- Impairment of logical thinking and abstract thought.
- Sequencing impaired – tasks cannot be performed in the correct order.

To help those with frontal lobe impairments, the following are suggested:

- As logic and the ability to plan are impaired, keep requests straightforward and literal.
- To compensate for the loss of sequencing, the person can be helped to complete tasks of daily living by placing items in the order required (eg, dressing, food preparation).
- Distraction can be the answer to perseveration. A noise, clapping or the sound of a bell is usually sufficient to restore the person to awareness. If the person is 'stuck' performing a task, a guiding hand will help.

The creation of individual rehabilitation programmes is probably one of the most demanding challenges for staff. When the neuropsychological basis of a person's difficulties is understood, and their problems are placed within the framework of an ecobehavioural analysis, an appropriate care plan can be introduced. Even a slight improvement in competence results in benefits not only for the person whose needs were previously unmet, but also for staff who feel an immense sense of achievement.

References

Bird M, Alexopoulos P & Adamowicz J, 1995, 'Success and Failure in Five Case Studies: Use of Cued Recall to Ameliorate Behaviour Problems in Senile Dementia', *International Journal of Geriatric Psychiatry,* 10, pp 305–11.

Bleathman C & Morton I, 1994, 'Psychological Treatments', Burns A & Levy R (eds), *Dementia,* Chapman & Hall Medical, London.

Dietch JT, Hewett LJ & Jones S, 1989, 'Adverse Effects of Reality Orientation', *Journal of the American Geriatric Society* 37, pp974–6.

Folsom JC, 1968, 'Reality Orientation Therapy for the Elderly Mental Patient', *Journal of Geriatric Psychiatry* 1, pp291–307.

Holden UP, 1990, 'Reality Orientation in the 1990s', in Stokes G & Goudie F (eds), *Working with Dementia*, Speechmark Publishing/Winslow Press, Bicester.

Hussian RA, 1981, *Geriatric Psychology: A Behavioural Perspective*, Van Nostrand Reinhold, New York.

Morton I & Bleathman C, 1988, 'Reality Orientation: Does It Matter Whether It's Tuesday or Friday?', *Nursing Times* 84(6), pp25–7.

Robertson IH, Halligan PW & Marshall JC, 1993, 'Prospects for the Rehabilitation of Unilateral Neglect', in Robertson IH & Marshall JC (eds), *Unilateral Neglect: Clinical Experimental Studies,* Laurence Erlbaum Associates, Hove.

Robertson IH, Tegner R, Tham K, Lo A & Nimmo-Smith, 1995, 'Sustained attention training for unilateral neglect. Theoretical and rehabilitation implications', *Journal of Clinical and Experimental Neuropsychology* 17, pp416–30.

Taulbee LR & Folsom JC, 1966, 'Reality Orientation for Geriatric Patients', *Hospital and Community Psychiatrist* 17, pp 133–5.

Woods RT, 1994, 'Reality Orientation', *Journal of Dementia Care* 2(2), pp24–5.

Further reading
Holden UP, 1995, *Ageing, Neuropsychology and the 'New' Dementias,* Chapman & Hall, London.
Sacks O, 1985, *The Man Who Mistook His Wife for a Hat,* Picador, London.

CHAPTER 10

Promoting Communication Skills with People who have Dementia

Pam Enderby

THE CAPACITY TO COMMUNICATE is the result of the ability to receive, retain, interpret, formulate, encode and express an idea; therefore cognition, sensory, neurosensory, neurophysiological and neuromotor systems are tested to the full in just this one activity. It is not surprising that people with dementia frequently have disorders of communication, considering the complexity of that process. These disorders may manifest themselves in different ways.

Many speech and language therapists have questioned whether they have a role to play in dementia. This chapter will argue that there is a role, but this should be carefully defined. Although specific expertise in this area is desirable, the general skills of a speech and language therapist can be of great assistance in the management of communication disorders related to dementia. Speech and language therapists traditionally undertake the roles of assessing, diagnosing, treating, educating and counselling all those with communication disorders, and certainly, although each aspect is modified in the area of dementia, they can still follow this pattern.

Assessment

There is no single assessment of speech and language that can describe, identify and discriminate the verbal and comprehension deficits associated with the different dementing conditions. It is possible that there will never be one. The speech and language assessment should be seen as part of the overall assessment of the client, contributing information to the general picture, which may or may not result in the diagnosis of dementia.

It is important to assess the whole communication process in order to identify both retained abilities and the kinds and frequencies of error. The way that a person with dementia attempts to repair communication difficulties can be indicative of the nature of the underlying problem. This may indicate awareness of communication breakdown; the degree of stress that this causes, and the other skills that are available to the person in order to remedy the situation.

Familiarity with the common problems associated with communication breakdowns will assist differential diagnosis. A brief summary of the main communication strategies used by normal elderly people, compared with three clinical conditions where communication problems are common, is presented in Table 10.1.

All readers will realise that it is not unusual for a person to present with more than one kind of problem. Thus an aphasic person may well be depressed, or a person with dementia may have some degree of additional specific aphasia; however, the general guidelines may be of assistance. Formal techniques, along with observation of, and participation in, conversation can elicit some of these behaviours, which will assist in identifying a diagnosis with regard to the type of communication breakdown. Those studying the language of persons with dementia see a pattern in its order of symptom presentation. The content and function of speech are often affected before the actual sounds of speech, while word order and grammar often remain relatively intact. A person with dementia may be able to speak more readily when asked direct questions, rather than being able to initiate conversation. The person with dementia may also have more difficulty with defining words, rather than naming objects.

Management of speech and language problems

One of the most vital roles regarding the management of people with dementia is easing the burden on carers by assisting them with techniques

Table 10.1 *Communication strategies and problems*

Communication associated with normal ageing
- Usually have good content of semantic memory (memory for meaning of words)
- Good inferencing and association
- A reduction in the generation of new ideas
- A delay in the access to vocabulary
- Grammar is well preserved
- Improvement of performance on language tasks, given time

Communication associated with aphasia
- Have difficulty with linguistic comprehension, particularly with words that occur less frequently and highly abstract language
- Have difficulty with linguistic expression
- Grammar and vocabulary are both vulnerable
- There is a willingness to participate in the communication and an attempt to repair errors in communication
- Non-linguistic expression and behaviour may be spared

Communication associated with depression
- Reduced motivation
- Poor concentration
- Slow responses
- Reduced responses
- May relate better to animals
- Variability of response
- Lack of gesture
- Little willingness to communicate

Communication associated with dementia
- The content of language is affected before the form
- Lack of sensitivity to context
- Breakdown in logical relationships
- Poor associative reasoning (problem-solving)
- Random topic initiation
- Grammar may be spared

that will facilitate better communication. The efficacy of speech and language therapy techniques with specific disorders associated with language dysfunction of people with dementia is still unclear. It would seem that teaching carers and relatives techniques that they can use in a consistent way has a more direct and long-lasting effect, and it may be that some techniques will help those who have, in addition to their dementia, other specific language disorders.

Ways of assisting comprehension

Frequently relatives will have modified their communication style over the period of time that communication has deteriorated. They will often know what works for them. Identifying these behaviours and making them explicit can be a useful way of acknowledging the expertise and experience of the carer and reinforcing the behaviour. Additionally, relatives and carers may find it helpful to use the following key points to improve communication, but therapists must be prepared to do more than just list these strategies. Role-playing, group practice and example are required to reinforce the new techniques.

• Reduce conflicting stimuli. Advise relatives to reduce distractions. For example, turn off the radio and television or, if the person with dementia is preoccupied (eg, fiddling with something on their lap), take their hands and speak directly facing them.
• It has been found to be helpful to raise the voice slightly at the beginning of a conversation to gain attention. It is also necessary to speak facing the person with dementia, ensuring that eye contact is kept.
• Slowing down speech slightly makes it easier for the person with dementia to process what is being said.
• Reduce the length of sentences and keep grammatical structures simple; ensure that one bit of information is given at a time.
• Use different ways of saying the same thing, so that the person with dementia is given the same piece of information in two or three different ways.
• Reduce possible confusions. Do not use terms like 'he' or 'she', but use the names of the people that you are talking about. Be specific with

regard to places and times, and give more prompts with regard to what you are talking about.

- Do not change the subject quickly. Introduce the topic that you are going to talk about carefully before extending the conversation. Use gesture if this will elaborate and not confuse. Point to pictures or objects when you talk about them, to help the person to remember.
- Be realistic: comprehension will be made worse if the patient is emotionally upset or tired. It is not worth trying to introduce important conversations at such times.
- Avoid open-ended questions, such as 'What shall we watch on television?' It may be better to ask 'Do you want to watch *this* or *this*?'
- Using a quiet, slow way of speaking can be soothing and reduce agitation. This can be useful even if the person is not understanding the context of what is being said. If the person with dementia has a very severe comprehension problem, intonation and tone of voice may be the main channel of communication.

Ways of assisting expression
- Encourage the person to communicate in whatever way is appropriate.
- Assist the person to control the conversation by reminding them of what they have said; for example, repeat what they have said immediately after them. You could change the words slightly if necessary.
- Encourage gesture, such as pointing or thumbs up.
- Listen to the intonation. This may be communicating more to you than the words themselves. You may gather from the intonation and the pitch of the voice whether the person with dementia is telling you about something happy or sad even if you cannot understand what the rest of the message is.
- Encourage the person with dementia to verbalise when they are doing something – for example, encourage them to say 'I'm going to have my dinner' just before mealtimes, or 'I'm going to walk down the garden' just before that activity. Include the person with dementia in conversation, in order to prevent isolation and withdrawal.
- Many people with dementia are happier with a familiar routine. If it is necessary to change a specific verbal behaviour, then a consistent

approach should be taken and this must be adhered to by all those caring for the person.

• Even when the person with dementia is talking what is apparent nonsense, do take some time to show you are attending and listening.

Personal biographies and their role in communication

There has been an increasing recognition that people with dementia bring to the illness their own experiences and histories in the form of a personal biography. These biographies, if known to those who care for them, can be used to trigger greater response by focusing on such topics. Also, painful or difficult subjects can be touched upon more sensitively if these are recognised. It is important that the biography contains information related to the names of pets, the names of family members, good friends, nicknames and so on, in order that these can be recognised if the person with dementia alludes to them. If the person with dementia has a severe communication problem, it is unlikely that he can assist the listener with appropriate context or background information. Therefore, it is essential that the listener is well informed in order to exploit any communication that is possible.

It is recommended that the personal biographies – in the form of logs – are developed with the individual and their families at an early point in their disease so that the many different caring professions that will come to have contact in the future can be appropriately informed and see the individual behind the disorder. Morton (Chapter 16) has more to say on communicating by means of reflective techniques with people who have severe language impairments.

One of the reasons why many relatives of persons with dementia are concerned that others cannot look after the person is that, because they have a shared history, frequently they are able to interpret the efforts of communication that may be misinterpreted by another.

Carer support groups

Many districts have support groups for the relatives of individuals with dementia, and the speech and language therapist can be very valuable in these groups. It is possible to do role-playing to establish the true nature of some of the ways of improving communication – for example, practising speaking slowly; looking at how to simplify language; really understanding what an open question is, and how to alter this. These are concrete activities that can be used as a task for the group to work on, and can in themselves promote some cohesion within the group.

Conclusion

The value of specific treatment of speech and language disorders in dementia remains a hotly debated issue. However, it is essential to remember that speech and language therapists, with their specialist skills and knowledge, have a role in the assessment, diagnosis and care of people with this disorder. Their training with regard to promoting and facilitating good communication is the very kind to which carers need access.

Further reading

Bayles K and Kaszniak A, 1987, *Communication and Cognition in Normal Ageing and Dementia*, Taylor & Francis, Philadelphia.

Kitwood T, 1997, *Dementia Reconsidered*, Open University Press, Buckingham.

Morton I, 2000, 'Just what is person-centred care?', *Journal of Dementia Care* 8(3), pp28–9.

CHAPTER 11

Responding to the Need to Toilet

Graham Stokes

GILLEARD (1984) FOUND THAT ONE of the most distressing behaviours families have to face is when a person with dementia starts to urinate in the 'wrong' places. It causes embarrassment and anger, and results in a heavy burden of intimate care. Yet why is it that such problems arise relatively early in some people, when for others it presents towards the end of a slow process of cognitive and behavioural decline? There is no simple answer to this question, for the achievement and maintenance of continence is a complex skill.

Toileting difficulty – not incontinence

When a person is found to be 'wet' or 'soiled' it is premature to automatically label them as incontinent. Incontinence denotes a failure of the controls associated with the normal storage of urine, and results in the involuntary passing of urine. It is therefore an explanation for impaired toileting, not a description of that behaviour.

A failure to toilet may also arise when bladder function is unimpaired. Stokes (1987) referred to this as inappropriate urinating. This is characterised by an awareness of a need to urinate that does not result in the acceptable passing of urine. It is thus premature to label an inability to toilet successfully as incontinence *unless* it is known that loss of or damaged bladder control is the *explanation*.

If we must label the behaviour of a person who wets or soils themselves, the term 'toileting difficulty' is preferable, for its usage logically leads on to the next question – 'why'? But before we examine possible explanations, it has to be acknowledged that to describe a person's behaviour as constituting a 'toileting difficulty' has, as yet, not offered us a precise and unambiguous description of behaviour. It remains an economical term open to misunderstanding and exploitation, for as a label it cannot define accurately the nature of the dependency.

Figure 11.1 shows how the tripartite model of assessment introduced by Stokes (1995a) is applied to the impairment of toileting skills. Commencing with the descriptive label, we progress to a definition that sets out the broad outline of the behaviour before moving on to a fine-grain description of what the person actually does.

The behavioural definition does not discriminate on the basis of presumed intent, but focuses on the deficient toileting actions. The

Label		Toileting difficulty
Behavioural definition:	**O P E R A T I O N A L D E F I N I T I O N**	The voiding of urine or faeces, either following an unsuccessful effort, or with no apparent attempt to employ an acceptable facility (eg, toilet, commode, urine bottle).
Behavioural characteristics:		Parcelling (eg, wrapping and concealing the evidence in drawers, cupboards, etc). Wetting or soiling clothes while sitting (passive). Wetting or soiling clothes while standing (active). Wetting or soiling the bed (passive). Using an inappropriate receptacle (eg, bin, fire bucket, plant, etc). Urinating against a wall. Smearing.

Figure 11.1 *The tripartite model of behavioural assessment*

behavioural characteristics reveal how the defined behaviour was acted out – for example, passive or active, discreet or invasive. 'Smearing' or 'parcelling' would be examples of invasive conduct. These descriptions are the bare bones of the methodology. Each practitioner will need to clothe the skeleton differently according to the individual toileting characteristics of the person with dementia. The practice of person-centred descriptions, rich in accurate detail, is known as 'pinpointing' – ie, pinpointing precisely the nature of their behaviour.

Toileting difficulty – a mosaic of explanation

To toilet appropriately a person requires the ability to negotiate a chain of discrete, but inter-related 'events' (both external and unobservable). These are described in Table 11.1.

The chain can break down at any point because of disease, disability, 'private events', which may include thoughts and beliefs, environmental factors or a mixture of all these.

While older adults may experience a need to pass urine with greater frequency, it is disturbance of the chain that results in a toileting difficulty.

Table 11.1 *The essential pathway to successful toileting*

1 Recognising the need to urinate and postponing within limits, the act of passing urine or faeces (failure = incontinence).
2 Being motivated to use the toilet.
3 Possessing the physical strength and steadiness to stand.
4 Possessing the mobility and confidence to cover the distance to the toilet and overcome any obstacles along the way (eg, floor coverings, stairs, out-stretched legs of others).
5 Maintaining goal-oriented behaviour.
6 Being able to locate the toilet (or acceptable alternative).
7 Perceiving and experiencing the toilet as accessible, safe, hygienic and private.
8 Possessing the dexterity and co-ordination to adjust clothing.
9 Initiating the act.

When seeking an explanation, it is essential to first discriminate between incontinence and unsuccessful performance following recognition of the need to urinate.

Incontinence: A person may soil themselves due to failure or impairment of bladder or bowel control so that involuntary voiding occurs. Such dysfunction may arise as a result of:

- A localised anatomical or physical abnormality. Incontinence may result from local disorders of the urinary tract. The manner of clinical presentation may result in a diagnosis of stress incontinence (involuntary loss of urine that occurs on physical exertion); urge incontinence (involuntary loss of urine associated with an uncontrollable desire to void that has not been anticipated), or overflow incontinence (the retention of urine with involuntary overflow). Consideration should also be given to the problems of urinary tract infection and constipation. Faecal incontinence may be caused by diabetes mellitus; age-related sphincter dysfunction; rectal prolapse, or be secondary to loose stools or constipation.
- Secondary nocturnal enuresis. After many years of complete control, a person may experience bed-wetting at night. This may be attributable to sleep weakening effective bladder control, or may indicate a more serious condition, such as heart failure.
- Loss of control. Incontinence can arise directly from the loss of learned bladder control due to cortical atrophy, while people with advanced dementia may have a neurologically disinhibited rectum (Barrett *et al*, 1990). Urinary incontinence may appear relatively early in the course of Pick's disease, as well as in sub-cortical dementia caused by multiple sclerosis.

Inappropriate urinating or bowel activity is characterised by an awareness of need that does not result in acceptable toileting behaviour.

- *Neuropsychological dysfunction* (for a description of terms see Chapter 9)
  - Expressive deficits will interfere with a person's capacity to communicate their need to toilet, and thus a request for assistance

to stand or locate the toilet may flounder on the rock of their disintegrated 'dementia speech'.

- Receptive dysfunction will mean that requests to toilet, or a query as to whether a person requires assistance, may not be understood and hence the need will remain unacknowledged.
- Visual agnosia may result in an inability to identify the toilet, so similar objects, such as a wash basin or bath may be used instead. A man I knew would urinate against white surfaces, including radiators, the side of a bath and in the corner of a room. Spatial agnosia will make it difficult, if not impossible for the person to find their way to the toilet.
- One-sided neglect means that a person will bump into things and fail to see objects on their 'blind' side. As they fail to appreciate anything to one side the implications for toileting are easy to appreciate.
- Apraxias interfere with toileting performance as order and sequencing are lost once the action is under voluntary control. A dressing apraxia renders the person well nigh incapable of achieving the appropriate arrangement of clothing prior to toileting. The result is soiled and wet clothing.
- Frontal lobe damage invariably results in impulsive, poorly reasoned actions that may result in a person defaecating in inappropriate places.

- *Disorientation*
  Toileting difficulties can arise following a move to new surroundings. A person who is unfamiliar with their environment may roam around the building searching for the toilet until they are compelled to urinate or defaecate inappropriately. It does not matter how often they are told, they will never learn, for their inability to store information works against the acquisition of information. Even when a person has lived for many years in the same house, the ravages of 'Ribot's Law' will result in the person with dementia becoming disorientated as their recent memories are lost.

- *Environment-dependent*
  Even when a person with dementia is aware of the location of the toilet, the design and layout of the building may make reaching it

difficult. The outcome may depend on the distance that has to be covered, and the strength and confidence the aged person possesses to avoid obstacles that may bar the way. Obstacles that may be obvious, such as stairs, steps and heavy doors, and those that may be not – for example, non-slip shiny floors that look wet and slippery to a pair of aged eyes, or a pattern on the floor or carpet that may suggest a step.

- *Loss of goal-directed behaviour*
  A person with dementia may get out of their chair with the objective of using the toilet, but then forget what they had intended to do. The fragmentation of experience may leave them walking apparently aimlessly with no obvious motive until the urge is so great they toilet wherever they may be.

- *Mobility and dexterity*
  Toileting difficulties may be the indirect consequence of physical disability. Despite being able to recognise the need to use the toilet, a person with dementia may be prevented from doing so because of unsteadiness while walking or standing, or because of slowness in moving. Alternatively, the person may reach the toilet in time, but have problems opening the door or adjusting their clothing because fine hand movements are compromised by the effects of arthritis or tremor associated with Parkinson's disease.

- *Depression*
  The appearance of a toileting difficulty may be the result of clinical depression. Older people with dementia are many more times more likely to suffer from depression than those who are younger, maybe by a factor of 10. Contrary to belief, loss of insight offers no protection. It is now widely accepted that depression in dementia warrants serious attention. When depressed, loss of interest, poor concentration, apathy and withdrawal combine to seriously interfere with toileting performance.

- *Apathy*
  Continence is an acquired habit, the motivation for which may diminish with loss of strength and stamina in old age. As life becomes

effortful, older adults conserve energy. For a minority, this may result in a disinclination to toilet appropriately.

- *Fear*
  A person with dementia may be frightened of falling, entering the unknown, negotiating stairs or becoming lost. It does not matter that we assess them as being competent; if a person feels frightened then that is what matters. Fear comes from within and is often impervious to the reassuring words of others. Fear may be exaggerated by sensory impairment or generated by perceptual distortions. Moniz-Cook *et al* (in press) describe the case of Jane, a woman who refused to enter the toilet, for to her it was 'crawling with worms'.

- *Embarrassment*
  Exposed to degrading care procedures; being too embarrassed to ask; fearful of humiliation if they were to wet or soil themselves on the way to the toilet, may result in a person discreetly wetting or soiling themselves. Unfortunately, their attempts to preserve dignity may result in condemnation and inevitable embarrassment. In advanced dementia, embarrassment may result in parcelling.

- *Curiosity*
  This explanation is especially pertinent at times of abnormal bowel movements – for example, constipation and diarrhoea, and may account for faecal smearing. Feeling uncomfortable, the person with dementia investigates to find out why. Having got faeces on their hands, they endeavour to clean themselves and remove the evidence of their actions. The fragmentation of experience and their enduring discomfort maintains their dysfunctional quest for knowledge.

- *Self-determination*
  The desire to exercise agency in intimate self-care may be so strong as to result in unsuccessful attempts to demonstrate independence, or as a consequence of unfailing pre-memorial knowledge a refusal to either ask for, or accept assistance.

- *Manipulation, attention-seeking and spite*
  The motivation is to get their own way, attract attention or retaliate. As cognitive capacity is required to set such objectives, this explanation is only valid at the beginnings of dementia, and invariably provides evidence of dysfunctional relationships.

- *Inadequate facilities*
  In communal arrangements (for example, day centres, residential homes, hospital wards), the number of toilets available may be inadequate to meet the needs of those who require them. This is especially pertinent at times of peak demand, say following mealtimes. The toilets may be difficult to enter, unclean or smell of stale urine; they may be poorly lit or lack adaptations to make them safe, or they may be too public. In their own right these failings do not result in inappropriate toileting. They do, however, discourage use and as a result they build in delay as the person embarks upon a potentially fruitless search for an acceptable toilet. The outcome is episodes of wetting and soiling.

- *Over-dependency*
  Over-concern by a family carer or the de-skilling effects of 'disempowerment', wherein a person is not allowed to use their remaining abilities, may lead to the premature loss of independent will and a regression to 'infantile' dependency.

- *Drug effects*
  Toileting difficulties may be a sign of drug side-effects. For example, they may be attributable to excessive drowsiness caused by tranquillisers, or an unwanted response of a person to diuretics. Bed-wetting and soiling at night may arise following the prescription of night-time sedation. Nasman *et al* (1993) associated faecal smearing with the use of benzodiazepines.

As can be seen, inappropriate toileting is by no means a straightforward problem to understand. Motivation and action will be enshrined within a person's biography and influenced by personal habit (see Stokes, 1995b; 1997). The range of explanation will also be affected by the progression of the presumptive disease. For example, motivational factors will be in part dependent on cognitive competence. Does the person possess insight? To what extent can they retain and recall experience and exercise reason?

Taxonomies of possible explanation enable us to understand the complex nature of behaviours. Patient-watching and listening have succeeded in opening our eyes and ears to a world to which the standard paradigm had failed to make reference. This same quest for understanding can inform and benefit everyday care practice. If we are watchful and creative in our thinking, we can brainstorm possible explanations for any behaviour that we face. The methodology may lack the scientific rigour of functional analysis, but what it brings is a dynamic approach to enquiry. For a description of the practice and benefits of 'creative brainstorming' see Stokes (2000).

When working with a person's toileting difficulty, the identification of cause may, however, be hindered by the hidden nature of the behaviour. It can be difficult to accurately identify an incident at the time of its occurrence if, for example, the person is either discreet, indifferent or unaware of their bodily functions. There is no simple solution to this difficulty. We need to be especially observant during the pursuit of understanding, and heed the clues that come from pinpointing the behavioural characteristics (for example, parcelling – embarrassment; passive wetting – incontinence, depression, or fear; smearing – curiosity; active wetting – apraxia, disorientation, or poor mobility; inappropriate receptacle – agnosia).

Finally, a person's behaviour is not only unique to them, but it can occur at different times for different reasons. To gain a genuine understanding of a person's behaviour it needs to be understood as it is occurring *now*. The example of Wendy (Case Study 11.1) illustrates how the reasons for a previous episode of toileting difficulty may have little bearing on the explanation for this or the next challenging incident.

Case Study 11.1 The trials of Wendy, aged 47 years, who has chronic-progressive multiple sclerosis

Wendy's husband could cope with much, but her wetting and soiling was beyond the pale. He would regularly ask whether she needed the toilet, invariably to be told no or to be met with silence. Then sometime later she would be found with clothes soiled, or there would be urine and faeces in the bed or on the toilet floor. Her rejection of his help angered him. Yet what infuriated him was that at the day centre her toileting difficulties were less severe. Her actions at home seemed deliberate. One day, having found his wife soiled on the way to the lavatory, just moments after having been asked whether she needed the toilet, he flew into a rage and grabbed hold of her. The casualty officer's report documented two broken fingers and a dislocated thumb.

There was no reason for Wendy's behaviour, instead there were reasons, some of which she found impossible to articulate:

- Damage sphincter control. Incontinence is a common feature of multiple sclerosis, and at times Wendy failed to acknowledge her need to toilet.
- Fatigue. Tiredness and loss of stamina significantly interfere with efficiency in daily life. Wendy would spend much of her time lying on the bed too tired to respond to her responsibilities and needs.
- Physical limitations on movement. Wendy had lost the sight in one eye and suffered from weakness and spasticity on her right side. As a result, her movements were slow and her co-ordination poor.
- Exaggerated forgetfulness. Wendy's dementia was mild, yet sufficient to compromise her memory and concentration. When somewhere new, she would sometimes struggle to locate the toilet even when reminded, but 'at the day care centre her toileting difficulties were less severe'.
- Depression. The most frequently observed emotional disturbance in multiple sclerosis is low mood. Wendy's family doctor had been treating her for depression for nearly two years, with little success.
- Forlorn attempts to maintain independence. Wendy was proud. She was determined to maintain her self-respect, even though her physical weakness rendered her increasingly dependent and likely to fail.
- Spite. Marital tensions pre-existed Wendy's multiple sclerosis. As her husband continued to live his life, often leaving her alone in the evening,

she would retaliate by soiling when he was out. This also enabled her to exercise a degree of control over her husband's activity.
- Embarrassment. In the absence of love and tenderness she found personal care at the hands of her husband awkward and embarrassing. She would rather try herself than experience the indignity of revealing her intimate needs to him.

Toileting difficulty – prevention

Multi-modal intervention is a preventative methodology that is integrated within the culture of care. It is a global environmental response to the challenge of 'toileting difficulty', helping many people to avoid the degrading experience of being found wet or soiled, by trawling the known causes and attempting to avoid, compensate or accommodate the reasons for their dysfunctional conduct.

On admission to new surroundings

To minimise the likelihood of adjustment anxieties and depression on admission to a residential home or hospital, a person with dementia should be welcomed with sensitivity. We should never underestimate the emotional upset and sense of threat that loss of home, broken relationships and the disruption of routines inevitably brings.

When a person with dementia demonstrates an inability to function in the most familiar environment available to them (ie, their home), we move them to a world that may in itself be truly fearful. They are taken away from familiar faces to live alongside people whom they do not see as being like them and who may, because of unexpected and inexplicable behaviours, be a potential source of insecurity and fear, not companionship.

To reduce the potential for distress and resigned indifference, there needs to be a sympathetic build-up to admission, with a phased entry to long-stay care as the ideal. All staff should see themselves as therapeutic workers, as involved with the internal world of their clients as with the external display of disability and dependency. This involves overcoming the barrier of dementia, and either through effective communication with the client or interviewing family and friends, learning about their habits, fears and insecurities as well as continuing strengths.

Effective welcoming procedures can prevent the onset of toileting difficulties that arise when we ignore the subjective world of feeling.

Medical and neuropsychological examination

Ensure that the person who arrives with toileting difficulties is examined by a GP so that reversible medical causes can be treated. Thereafter, routine health screening should be a feature of later life. This is particularly important where people with dementia are concerned, as they are often unable to express their health needs. All drugs being taken should be regularly reviewed.

Neuropsychological examination will help to identify the existence of focal brain damage and the severity of memory impairment. How we may assist people with such brain dysfunction is discussed in Chapter 9.

Mobility and sensory impairments

If someone's mobility needs to be improved, is the involvement of a physiotherapist or chiropodist required? Would walking aids be of use? Is there a need to correct, or compensate for, visual deficits? If a confused elderly person wears glasses, do not assume automatically that these meet their current requirements.

Diet

To prevent constipation, the elderly person's diet requires sufficient roughage. Regular consumption of fruit, vegetables, wholemeal bread and high-fibre breakfast cereals is recommended. Is there a need to request the assistance of a dietician?

Infection control

To prevent episodes of diarrhoea, infection control procedures need to be in place and, most importantly, practised with diligence.

Fluids

Drinking habits should always be observed as there is a need for an adequate daily fluid intake. Some people may drink excessively, while others drink too little. If necessary, keep an accurate record of intake and output.

Night-time routines

Caregivers need to ensure that people pass urine before going to bed, unless a person's habits suggest an alternative routine. During the night, in residential and nursing home settings, regularly check whether those who are awake want to use the toilet.

The decision to wake people who regularly wet the bed so that they can pass urine appropriately must be considered alongside the possible resulting problems of disorientation, resistance and daytime fatigue. I had a client who was given her night-time sedation at 8pm, disturbed at 10pm to take anti-convulsant medication, and then awakened at 2 am and 6 am to check whether her bed was wet. Was it any wonder that throughout the day she regularly wet herself as she dozed in her chair?

The provision of care

Sometimes requests to be toileted are 'false alarms' – the person fails to perform when taken to the toilet. This often happens at busy times on a ward or unit, or when a carer at home is occupied elsewhere, and it can try a caregiver's patience. But it may be someone's desperate effort to ensure they never experience the indignity of wetting or soiling themselves. The person is not simply to be dismissed as a nuisance, but should be seen as a person with a regard for hygiene and self-respect who feels their needs may be ignored because their carers are so busy.

In residential homes, sometimes the issue is not excessive demands, but a reluctance to ask. Where staff do not wear uniforms, be aware that a resident may be too embarrassed to request assistance in case they mistakenly seek help from a visitor. Also bear in mind that an elderly man may be reluctant to ask for help with toileting from young female members of staff.

It is important that when a person who is known to be unable to toilet themselves asks for assistance, it is a disservice to the individual to either ignore that person's requests because they are equated with attention-seeking, or to introduce unnecessary delay that leads to avoidable and embarrassing incidents of inappropriate urinating. I have never forgotten the findings of our 'back in a minute' study on a hospital ward – they rarely returned, and never within 60 seconds!

If people with dementia are not allowed to exercise their toileting skills because standards of efficiency, cleanliness and hygiene take on a disproportionate importance for caregivers, there will be an unnecessary increase in dependence as individuals lose the motivation to care for themselves. Give them as much responsibility for their own care as is realistic. Whether the person is in their own home or in other accommodation they should not be hurried as they attempt to maintain independence. In the short term, carers may see this as a time-consuming activity, but overall the benefits of maintaining independence, even for a few months, outweigh the burden of escalating dependence.

Dressing

A person's dressing ability should be assessed and, if necessary, practice in dressing skills should be provided. It may be advantageous to arrange for clothing adaptions. Velcro fastenings to replace buttons can assist people who have toileting difficulties because of dressing problems. Always remember, however, that normal clothing should be worn, because personal appearance plays a large part in determining how others react, and this in turn influences self-respect.

Interior design and layout

Through the use of signs, symbols, colour-coding and 'pathfinder' information, elderly people with memory damage can be helped to locate the toilet. The use of night lights in the toilet and approach areas not only helps to reduce fear and disorientation, but it also means that accidents are less likely.

In residential and hospital settings there must not only be an adequate number of toilets, but toilet facilities should be readily accessible at all times. They should be near (within approximately 10 to 15 metres), and the approach obstacle-free, well lit and safe. It is always the case that people who sit furthest away from the toilets display the greatest evidence of 'incontinence'.

All doors – whether the exit from a lounge, or the entrance to the toilet – should be easy to open and wide enough to allow entry using a walking frame. They should not be heavy, as this will present a formidable barrier to progress. Nor should they be spring-loaded, as there is a risk of them rebounding on slow-moving residents passing through.

The toilet seat should be sufficiently high to make it easy for residents to get up and down. Handrails at either side of the toilet for extra support are advisable. The toilet area should be private, warm and have plenty of room for manoeuvring walking aids. To protect dignity, the toilet should not be sited opposite the door, nor should toilet doors be left wide open in order to aid observation. A call system by the toilet creates a sense of confidence.

Toileting difficulty – resolution

Even in supportive surroundings, toileting difficulties can arise. However, just because the chain of adaptive behaviour snaps we do not disempower by taking over, submerging people in care, and creating 'excess disabilities'. Instead, we identify where the person has difficulty and embark upon an individual plan of action.

If dysfunctional behaviour can be addressed through change within the person, goal-planning is the recommended option (Barrowclough & Fleming, 1986). Goal-planning is a structured approach that draws upon a person's remaining strengths (ie, what they can do, like to do, and who will be willing to help them), in order to help and motivate them toward tackling their difficulties and meeting their needs. Yet we often need to be helped to see strengths in people, for it is often easier to see weakness (she can't walk far) rather than strength (she can still walk from her bedroom to the toilet).

Goudie (1990) describes how realistic goal plans are devised (realistic in terms of the person's residual abilities and what the care setting can offer), and how these address in a positive way key questions such as 'what will the person do'; 'who will they do it with'; 'how will they do it'? We accept that for many people goals will be limited in ambition. For example, if a person is no longer aware of or motivated to use the toiletm our intervention may take the form of building on the strengths that remain and introducing an individualised approach such as daytime habit retraining or patterned urge response toileting (PURT) (Colling *et al*, 1992).

Daytime habit retraining

When a person's pattern of toileting guides the programme it is known as habit retraining. As inflexible toileting procedures should not be imposed upon people in care who reveal predictable toileting needs, this approach has much to recommend it. It can be an effective strategy to employ in those cases where a toileting difficulty arises because of, for example, demotivation or disability, which prevent independent toileting ever being a realistic goal.

The objective is to remind the person to void at intervals that will anticipate incidents of wetting or soiling, in order to produce an acceptable toileting rhythm.

In the beginning, as with patterned urge response toileting (PURT), a person is checked initially at fixed intervals – say every two hours to establish whether they are wet, soiled or dry. They are then prompted and assisted to use the toilet. The outcome of this intervention is recorded on a habit retraining assessment chart, which can take the form of the example below.

Habit Retraining Assessment Chart

TIME	am							pm						
Day	Date	8.00	9.00	10.00	11.00	12.00	1.00	2.00	3.00	4.00	5.00	6.00	7.00	8.00	9.00
		C T	C T	C T	C T	C T	C T	C T	C T	C T	C T	C T	C T	C T	C T

KEY	State of resident (C)	Result of toileting (T)
C = Check square	D = Dry	Passed faeces = Blue
T = Toilet use dot	W = Wet	Passed urine = Yellow
	S = Soiled	No use = Red star
		Refused = Oblique line (/)

Information is recorded on a person's state and whether the prompt resulted in toilet use. As it is desirable to keep to a minimum the number of occasions when voiding does not occur, there is a need to identify those visits to the toilet that were unnecessary.

If a pattern is revealed over a number of days (at least three), then the person is suitable for habit retraining. At those times when the person was found to be consistently soiled or wet, adjustments are made to the schedule, so they are accompanied to the toilet before voiding occurs. Similarly, visits to the toilet may be discontinued if a person has regularly failed to void when taken to the toilet. In this way the programme is amended according to the person's needs.

For example, the following results may be obtained:

	8.00 am	10.00 am	12.00 noon	2.00 pm	4.00 pm	6.00 pm	8.00 pm
Check	Wet	Wet	Dry	Dry	Soiled	Wet	Dry
Toilet use	Yes	No	Yes	No	No	Yes	Yes

Observation has revealed episodes of wetting and soiling at 8.00 am, 10.00 am, 4.00 pm and 6.00 pm, and non-usage of the toilet at 10.00 am, 2.00 pm, and 4.00 pm.

To pre-empt the passing of urine and faeces, the schedule is adjusted so that toilet prompts take place half an hour earlier than the original check times when the person was discovered wet or soiled. In addition, those checks when the person was found to be dry, but the prompt to use the toilet did *not* result in usage, are now discontinued.

The resulting schedule of toilet prompts, is as follows: 7.30 am, 9.30 am, 12.00 noon, 3.30 pm, 5.30 pm and 8.00 pm.

As you can see, the number of toilet visits has been reduced to six from the original seven. So not only does this procedure benefit the person, who is saved the indignity of unnecessary toileting, it also allows for a more efficient use of caregiver time.

The final stage in habit retraining is to extend the intervals between prompts by 15 minutes, until three-hourly intervals are established throughout the day. Following a successful outcome to this stage, prompted toileting will have been markedly reduced.

As a result of adjusting and extending the time between toileting prompts, so that voiding is postponed for as long as possible, a new pattern of predictable need is established, which enables the person with dementia to remain dry and clean, as well as avoiding fruitless journeys to the toilet.

When working with a person who has the capacity to retain the benefits of experience (the beginnings of dementia), yet is lacking motivation, backward chaining can be an effective response to the need to toilet.

Backward chaining – on the path to 'rementia'

This method of relearning starts at the end of the sequence of toileting behaviours. We establish the final step first, and only then go on to the preceding link in the chain. For example, you can concentrate initially on the person's ability to rearrange clothing after toilet use. Once practice in this dressing skill has established the behaviour, focus on the act of voiding while on the toilet. Eventually you direct your intervention toward the 'approach' behaviours, such as finding the way to the toilet; getting up and walking to the toilet, and ultimately making the decision to go to the toilet when necessary. Each component part of the chain of toileting skills can be relearned in this way. Learning is encouraged by the use of social reinforcers (these may be verbal, as in a remark of gentle praise, or physical, as a squeeze of the hand).

The advantage of backward chaining is that the completion of the chain possesses the reward of fulfilment. As such, concentrating on the skills closest to completion motivates relearning. Once acquired, preceding steps can be learned with the knowledge that the chain can be completed. This again serves to encourage the goal of 'rementia'.

Conclusion

By providing a global response to toileting difficulties, the multi-modal approach has shown itself to be a successful therapeutic strategy, helping many people avoid the degrading experience of being found wet and soiled. However, it will not meet the needs of all people. For some, individualised goal planning may be the most effective means of reducing dependency, by motivating and helping people to do as much for themselves as possible for as long as possible.

For those people at the end stage of dementia, all will have lost bladder and bowel control. To help them stay clean and dry, either a rigid toileting regime implemented at regular intervals throughout the day or, as a last resort, the introduction of continence aids is advised. It should always be remembered, however, that people with severe dementia will be unaware of their own disabilities and weaknesses, and thus may reject assistance as both unnecessary and unwelcome. At these times a person is not to be seen as awkward, but as an individual whose plight deserves to be met with sensitivity and empathy.

References

Barrett JA, Brocklehurst JC, Kiff ES, Ferguson G, & Faragher EB, 1990, 'Rectal Motility Studies in Geriatric Patients with Faecal Incontinence', *Age and Ageing* 19, pp311–17.

Barrowclough C & Fleming I, 1986, *Goal Planning with Elderly People,* Manchester University Press, Manchester.

Colling J, Ouslander J, Hadley BJ, Eish J & Campbell E, 1992, 'The Effects of Patterned Urge-Response Toileting (PURT) on Urinary Incontinence Among Nursing Home Residents', *Journal of the American Geriatrics Society* 40(2), pp135–41.

Gilleard CJ, 1984, *Living with Dementia,* Croom Helm, London.

Goudie F, 1990, 'Goal Planning: Towards Meeting Individual Needs', in Stokes G & Goudie F (eds), *Working with Dementia*, Speechmark Publishing/Winslow Press, Bicester.

Moniz-Cook E, Stokes G & Agar S, in press, 'Difficult Behaviour and Dementia in Nursing Homes: Five Cases of Psychosocial Intervention', *International Journal of Clinical Psychology and Psychotherapy.*

Nasman B, Bucht G, Eriksson S & Sandman PO, 1993, 'Behavioural Symptoms in the Institutionalised Elderly – Relationship to Dementia', *International Journal of Geriatric Psychiatry* 8, pp843–9.

Stokes G, 1987, *Common problems with the Elderly Confused: Incontinence and Inappropriate Urinating*, Speechmark Publishing/Winslow Press, Bicester.

Stokes G, 1995a, 'Incontinent or Not? Don't Label: Describe and Assess', *Journal of Dementia Care* 3(1), pp 20–21.

Stokes G, 1995b, 'Incontinent or Not? Person First, Dementia Second', *Journal of Dementia Care* 3(2), pp20–21.

Stokes G, 1997, 'Reacting to a Real Threat', *Journal of Dementia Care* 5(1), pp14–15.

Stokes G, 2000, *Challenging Behaviour in Dementia*, Speechmark Publishing/Winslow Press, Bicester.

CHAPTER 12

Activity, Occupation and Stimulation

Tessa Perrin

L ET ME BEGIN THIS CHAPTER by asking a question. Have you ever thought about the difference between activity and occupation? I hadn't (despite the fact that I have been an occupational therapist for a long time and ought to know better) until I bothered to look it up in the dictionary not so long ago. I discovered that there is a big difference. The word activity very simply means 'doing things', nothing more, nothing less. Occupation, on the other hand, is a broad concept which has to do with taking hold or seizing the thing that you want, losing yourself in the satisfaction of it and making it very personally yours. A big difference, and a difference to be found not only in the words of the dictionary, but also in the policies and practices of care settings for older people. Over the years, many care settings have been content simply to 'do things' – in other words, to provide a fairly random regime of activities and entertainment for people to take or leave as they wish. Activity has commonly been understood as 'the bingo session', 'the reminiscence group' or 'the outing'. Activity provision has not been a priority and has attracted little resourcing in the way of personnel, training or finance. Such a picture is still common to many care settings today.

But this is no longer good enough. We are now much more aware than we used to be of the importance of occupation in healthcare. We know from research that engaging in occupation is critical to physical and psychological health and wellbeing. We also know that doing any old activity is not enough; it might well keep us busy, but it won't necessarily improve our health or our sense of wellbeing. For a significant impact on health and wellbeing we need to find and give ourselves to those pursuits that have meaning, and are pleasurable and absorbing. This is as true for you and me as it is for our elderly client, and puts our activity provision in care settings under rather a different light. For the thing that is meaningful, pleasurable and absorbing for me is unlikely to hold the same qualities for you. It might, but it might not, for occupation is a highly individual thing. What is interesting and stimulating to one can be mind-numbingly boring to another. What is rewarding, satisfying and therefore therapeutic to this person may be distasteful, frustrating and counter-productive to that person. Therefore, for a care setting simply to provide an arbitrary programme of group activities and entertainments is not enough. These have their place, but if what we are about is truly individualised person-centred care, we need to take a fresh look at our practice.

We are occupational beings, and we each have a unique occupational identity. Any care regime that fails to embrace this concept and make provision for individual occupational need cannot call itself truly person-centred. Our starting point, then, is to build a full and detailed occupational profile, drawn where possible from our clients themselves, but also from family, friends, home carers and, of course, from our own direct observations of our client in the care setting. Questions we need to ask are:

- With what things did this person fill their life?
- Which of these things would they have called work, and which leisure?
- What were their daily routines and habits?
- What were their main roles in life?
- Of the things with which they filled their life, what can they still do? What do they still like/want to do? What things have they now rejected?

Let us make no mistake about this. We are not talking here about filling in a brief form with sections on hobbies and interests. We don't just want to know if they went to bingo every Tuesday, or like Bing Crosby, or what television programmes they watch. People are occupied from the moment they get up in the morning till the time they go to bed at night. We want the whole picture of their occupational life, not just the things they once used to fill in the gaps between work and family. Only when we have this kind of information can we start to work with our client to develop that personalised programme of daily activities that is just right for them. This is the starting point of any therapeutic relationship. But when our client has dementia, the need for careful assessment is even more important, for the person with dementia cannot always tell us how they like to spend their day, or what they want to do. We therefore need to be particularly cautious in our approach. I believe that many of us have caused damage to our clients in the past, not intentionally, but simply because we have failed to understand the effects of their disability on the things they do, and placed them in situations that are too demanding for their level of ability. Mrs Morris (Case Study 12.1) is a good illustration of this.

Case Study 12.1 Mrs Morris starts to laugh

Mrs Morris used to attend a day centre where I once worked. She had quite a severe impairment, although you wouldn't know it to look at her – she was always immaculately turned out, due to the assistance of her daughter, with whom she lived. But she never spoke; never did anything in fact. She would arrive at the day centre, sit, look miserable and go home; arrive the next day, sit, look miserable and go home. It was always the same – until the day I took a large, soft, yellow beach-ball into the centre. She was transformed. She would throw, catch and kick whenever the ball came in her direction. She started to smile and laugh and engage others in eye contact. She actually got out of her chair from time to time to fetch the ball, and sometimes a healthy bit of competition would spice up the occasion.

It was quite by chance that we discovered Mrs Morris' simple pleasure in ball and balloon games. At the time I thought no more of it, beyond being glad to have found something that made her day a little more worthwhile. But looking back, I understand now that all our previous attempts to engage Mrs Morris had been inappropriate, and their inappropriateness had probably served only to deepen the depression and anxiety that were so much a part of her habitual demeanour. We had been working very hard to draw her into the general activities of the group – quizzes, discussions, crafts. Most clients in the group were more able than Mrs Morris and enjoyed such activities, and with the best will in the world we wanted her to share in that. But unwittingly we were actually making things worse for her, for Mrs Morris had gone well beyond the point where she could comfortably participate in activities of this kind, which require quite sophisticated intellectual, verbal and manual skills. I believe that at some level Mrs Morris knew and felt bad that she could no longer function as she once could. With the ball game, we happened by chance to get that all-important 'fit' between ability and activity; we had matched a sensory-motor activity to a lady who was now functioning predominantly at a sensory-motor level of ability. That is, having lost most of her intellectual, daily living and social skills through her dementia, she was operating from those she had left, the elementary, basic skills upon which all others are built.

Our work with Mrs Morris had a positive outcome and we were glad for that, but had we known what we know now, I think we could have saved her a lot of distress along the way. What we have now, at the time of writing, is the beginning of a theoretical underpinning to our work in activities and dementia – a guideline to help us to direct our interventions to therapeutic effect. We no longer have to be quite so random or hit and miss in our approach to activities as we have been in the past. We no longer have any excuse for just 'doing things', engaging in any activity because any activity has to be better than none.

Perrin and May (1999) hold the opinion that dementia is most helpfully understood as a sort of 'return journey' back through the developmental milestones that we go through in the course of our childhood development. As children and young people, we develop our skills in a sequential fashion; in other words, we cannot acquire this skill until we have first acquired a more basic skill. We might imagine our development as the building of a wall: the foundations are laid first; then the first row of bricks; then the second, and so on. It would be impossible to build from the top down. Broadly speaking, this is how we all mature to the full complement of the skills required to equip us for independent living. Using the same analogy, we might understand dementia as the gradual dismantling of the wall; the top bricks that were laid last come off first; the foundations that were laid first are retained longest.

The return journey is unique in every case, of course, but it can be a helpful analogy to look at the skill level of a child or young person and at the activities that they can enjoy in the context of those skills. For if a person with dementia has returned to an earlier, more elementary, level of function, we should consider the possibility that they might enjoy activities of the kind that engage a young person.

This idea, with its implications of a 'return to childhood', is a challenging one for some, but it is one we must consider. There is no suggestion here of treating people in any kind of demeaning or infantilising way. Of course we treat people as adults, with the courtesy and sensitivity with which we ourselves would wish to be treated. But recognising that people are functioning at an earlier developmental level releases us to understand that people now do things differently and, if we are to get that 'fit' between ability and activity, we must accommodate that 'differentness'. 'Fit' will almost invariably manifest itself in our client in a clear expression of engagement, absorption, pleasure and satisfaction, and that, of course, is our yardstick for the measure of any intervention. What we seek is wellbeing – wellbeing through occupation – and if our interventions are not eliciting wellbeing, we need to think again.

The guideline to illustrate the effects of the return journey and possible occupational interventions is outlined in schematic form in Figure 12.1.

We need to bear in mind that this is not an assessment tool. It is a guideline only – a schema for helping us to understand a situation and plan a course of action. We need to remember two things as a rule of thumb when considering applying this schema to our planning:

1 A person who has returned to a given level of ability is most likely to accommodate, use and enjoy the activities designated *at that level*. Activities at a *later* developmental level are likely to be experienced as too demanding, and therefore stressful.
2 We also need to consider that a person might appreciate – even relish – some of the activities designated at an *earlier* developmental level.

Figure 12.1 *Wellbeing through occupation (Adapted from Perrin T & May H, 1999)*

Developmental stage	Reflective phase (Early dementia)	The symbolic phase (early to middle dementia)	The sensory-motor phase (middle to late dementia)	The reflex phase (Late dementia)
Skills	Thought processes are complex and fluid. We can sort and weigh information, deal with multiple stimuli, make decisions, express choices, form opinions. We can look back, plan ahead, think beyond our own four walls into the world of others. We have the optimum capacity for making relationships of different kinds and at different levels of intimacy.	Thought processes are becoming more concrete. We can deal with fewer and fewer stimuli and we cannot think in concepts and abstracts. We are losing a sense of the wider environment – peripheral places, people and projects are beginning to fade. Relationships are beginning to change. Symbols, those mental images such as memories and feelings, are pre-eminent.	The ability to engage with the world in language is mostly gone. Relationships have changed. The world now centres around self, and the needs and concerns of others are not appreciated. In the absence of intellectual, social and daily living skills, the world is understood and experienced primarily through the sensory and motor mechanisms of the body.	Intentional actions are mostly gone. Repetitive single-step actions appear comforting. Ultimately only reflex and imitative responses to stimuli are evident.

Developmental stage	Reflective phase (early dementia)	The symbolic phase (early to middle dementia)	The sensory-motor phase (middle to late dementia)	The reflex phase (Late dementia)
Nature of activity	We can accommodate activities structured around rules, sequences and goals. We often seek activity that involves collaboration with others, and enjoy a competitive element.	Our ability to deal with rules, goals and competition is declining. Working alongside others is more comfortable than working in cooperation. Symbolic activities that centre around the pictures and feelings of long-term memories and relationships are key.	Activities that demand structured thought and language are usually rejected. Activities involving physical, motor skills and sensory appreciation are usually welcomed.	Conventional activities have ceased, but actions remain. Only one-to-one engagement is possible, and that mostly in terms of being done to rather than independent doing.
Suitable activities	Games Sports Quizzes Discussions Crafts End-product tasks	Music Dance Art and pottery Movement Drama Reminiscence Story-telling Spiritual activity	Movement and exercise Multi-sensory environments Massage One-step cooking tasks One-step gardening tasks Pet animals Stacking and folding Dolls and soft toys Balls/bubbles/balloons	Smiling Singing Stroking Rocking Holding Cuddling

These will generally not exert undue demand, and who among us has not enjoyed the pure sensory-motor pleasure (and the 'undemandingness') of a massage, a cuddle of a warm puppy, or a silly balloon game at the Christmas party? We need to exercise sensitivity and some caution here, for we do not wish to deskill or demean a person, but if we use as our yardstick evidence of pleasure and satisfaction – the smile, the engagement, the eye contact, the shared humour – these things will guide us and ensure that we are not going too far wrong.

We need to say a word here about the activities categorised in the schema as symbolic, for these are something of an exception to the rule of thumb. Many symbolic activities may be appreciated across all levels of decline, even into late dementia, because they are activities that centre around feelings and inner pictures, images and memories, some of which may be retained well into late dementia; and, of course, those of us on the outside will never know quite how much is retained on the inside.

This schema, then, is our first point of reference in establishing that 'fit' we have spoken of above. Beyond that, particularly in later dementia, it is likely to be a matter of trial and error – a testing out of this activity and that until we find those to which our client responds positively. We are not looking simply for engagement. The fact that someone simply does what we ask; 'does things' for the sake of it or to please us, is not sufficient. We need to revisit our earlier definition; we want evidence that somebody has picked up this activity and made it their own; that it absorbs and gives them pleasure; that they can lose themselves in it; that they can express themselves through it, and initiate engagement of their own accord (Case Study 12.2).

Case Study 12.2 Frank becomes assistant ward domestic

Frank was a man in early dementia, having some respite time on a continuing care ward. He didn't have much useful language left, but he was fit, active and energetic. Quite of his own accord he took on the role of assistant ward domestic, and he expressed real concern that the lady who was employed as the domestic should have to carry out heavy, dirty tasks such as carrying buckets and mopping floors (clearly, he was also a gentleman!). I have never seen a man with dementia work as Frank worked. The domestic actually couldn't mop a floor if Frank was around because he would literally wrest the mop and bucket from her. While she was working he couldn't rest, sometimes even leaving his pudding uneaten on the table to assist her as she worked through the residents' lunch-time.

Using the schema outlined above, Frank would have slotted into the 'reflective' category; quite damaged in some respects, but still able to understand sequences of a process, to work towards a goal, to use tools appropriately, and to accomplish a task with some manual dexterity. Frank did other things too, but this he loved, made his own and entered into body and soul. A perfect 'fit'!

Case Study 12.3 Madeleine enjoys a hand massage

Madeleine was in late dementia, recliner-chair-bound, with neither language nor speech and little independent action. I watched one day as the visiting aromatherapist gave her a hand massage. She sat low at Madeleine's side, spread a towel on her lap and massaged one hand and then the other with some perfumed oil. She spoke gently to Madeleine on and off throughout, of nothing in particular, and not minding that Madeleine couldn't reply. What struck me as I watched was the depth and commitment of Madeleine's engagement with the activity. She wasn't 'doing' to be sure; she was 'being done to'. But nevertheless her engagement was total. Madeleine could still do two things: she could smile and she could engage eye contact – and she did both throughout. Every time the therapist lifted her eyes from the massage and caught Madeleine's, Madeleine would beam; radiant was the word that came to mind. In fact, such was the intimacy of relationship that appeared to develop, that I felt intrusive just sitting watching.

People often say that those with advanced dementia can't or don't 'do' anything any more. Actually, this is true of very few. Madeleine (Case Study 12.3) was in the reflex phase of dementia and, despite the severity of her disabililty, she was able to appreciate some sensory stimuli and actively to enjoy them. I believe she was, in her own self-contained way, every bit as enthused and engaged as Frank. Another perfect 'fit'.

We should not expect, of course, that everybody will respond with such vitality, nor that such a commitment to engagement can always be sustained for long periods. Quite apart from anything else, the more advanced the dementia, the less able the person is to engage in activity without the intervention of the carer; and if we are concerned about quality dementia care, we must acknowledge that it is inescapably time-consuming. But let us take a lead from our own experience. Much of our day-to-day life is in the 'doing of things', tasks and routines that must be done, but which do not enthuse or delight us. But without the punctuation of those times with episodes of comfort and pleasure in which we are taken out of the humdrum, life would be grey indeed. Such times lift us and sustain us. It is no different for the person with dementia.

Most of us aspire towards a culture of care in which we have the luxury of time for those we care for, unhindered and uninterrupted. That is likely to be a long time coming. Until it does, our task is to provide interludes of occupation for each individual. The activity programme, the entertainments, the outings, these all have their place; we should not dismiss them. But let us ensure that they do not stand in the way of a truly person-centred plan of occupation. Health and wellbeing depend on it.

References
Perrin T & May H, 1999, *Wellbeing in Dementia: An Occupational Approach for Therapists and Carers*, Churchill Livingstone.
Clarke A, Hollands J & Smith J, 1996, *Windows to a Damaged World*, Counsel and Care.
Csikszentmihalyi M, 1975, *Beyond Boredom and Anxiety*, Jossey-Bass, California.
Csikszentmihalyi M, 1992, *Flow: The Psychology of Happiness*, Rider, London.

Further reading
Hurtley R & Wenborn J, 2000, *The Successful Activity Co-ordinator's Handbook*, Age Concern.

PART 4

CHALLENGING BEHAVIOUR

CHAPTER 13

Working with Aggression: Prevention and Intervention

Graham Stokes

CHALLENGING BEHAVIOUR PLACES considerable demands on the tolerance, resilience and coping abilities of both families and care staff. Agitation, withdrawal, aggression, wandering, confusion, noise-making and demandingness are the most common reasons for treatment with psychotropic medication and hospitalisation. Families are more likely to seek help because of crises created by behavioural disturbances than by intellectual impairment itself. The capacity of family carers to cope dissolves in the face of challenging behaviour, not simply because of the level of skill required to care for somebody who is as likely to hit you as welcome you, but because the appearance of disruptive behaviour is often taken as testimony that they are no longer caring for the person once 'known and loved'. At such times, can we reasonably expect them to devote time and energy (the so-called '36-hour day') to caring for this stranger, or maybe not a stranger?

One of the most serious challenging behaviours associated with dementia is aggression, yet the question of what to label as aggressive behaviour is by no means straightforward.

In a study that associated violence with dementia, Shah (1992) defines violence 'as any act of physical aggression involving physical contact.' The levels of violence observed were low, and the severity of injury from assaults mild. Clearly, the high prevalence of aggression in dementia is the consequence of behaviour other than physical assault. Ware *et al* (1990) reported that aggressive behaviour caused great distress to carers despite the absence of physical violence. Several researchers (eg, Shah, 1991) believe that the under-reporting of aggressive behaviour is in part the result of the term being so ill-defined, and that observer perception and tolerance of threat dominate reporting behaviour (see Inness, 1998). A study by Dean *et al* (1993) noted that an increase in 'aggressivity' reported by staff was accounted for by residents being 'better able to express themselves and make demands.'

Being uncooperative or resisting help (for example, pushing people away when they offer assistance), irritability and verbal abuse are the most common kinds of aggressive behaviour (Patel & Hope, 1992). When physical aggression is observed it manifests itself most commonly as biting, scratching, kicking and hitting, which on occasions can be dangerous (Ware *et al*, 1990). Destructive acts and sexual aggression are rare.

Operational definition

Behavioural definition
Aggressive behaviour is injurious conduct involving the delivery of verbal abuse, or the threat or actual act of physical assault, spite, or destruction of property, which is unquestionably non-accidental.

Behavioural characteristics

Spitting	Tripping	Damage to property
Hitting	Pinching	Destroying property
Biting	Pushing	
Slapping	Nudging	
Scratching	Jabbing with elbow	Swearing
Kicking		Insults
Using an object to hit another	Threatening to harm	Being sarcastic and derogatory
Physical resistance to care		Yelling at another
		Blaming and accusing

The characteristics incorporated within the definition *exclude*:

- Irritability – an emotional state that is ill-defined and questionably observed
- Being uncooperative – this may represent an unwillingness that is a legitimate act of assertiveness and thus to be respected
- Self-harm – an act worthy of consideration in its own right.

An accurate and agreed definition of aggressive behaviour is essential for appropriate understanding and intervention. If the assessment is inadequate, the potential outcomes are misguided labelling, ill-advised interventions and the inappropriate use of psychotropic medication.

Aggression – common explanations

Seeking explanations for aggressive behaviour so often involves looking at the aggressor not as the culprit but as a person who has been unintentionally provoked. Hence, it is not for them to change, but for us to do so.

Defensive behaviour

Aggression may be a defensive reaction to the threat of intrusion of personal space. Providing assistance in basic self-care tasks may be resisted as the purpose is not understood and carers are not recognised.

The interrelated issues are:

1 Entering an individual's personal space without invitation or explanation (or if one is provided it is inadequate, for it is ambiguous; fails to appreciate that the person may be hard of hearing; does not take into account their receptive difficulties, or is not repeated).
2 Delivering 'hands-on' intimate care once in their personal space to a person who is unable to know their dependency needs.
3 Failing to acknowledge that we are obscured by a mist of disorientation. Our intentions are unknown and our credibility is minimal: for a while we know who we are and what we are doing, they rarely, and then only fleetingly, ever do.

The outcome has been referred to as 'aggressive resistance' (Hope *et al*, 1997).

Failure of competence

With insight remaining, attempts to help the person with activities of daily living may be unwelcome. They are explicit evidence of incompetence and, as such, help may be resisted and abuse may dominate the attempted episode of care.

Similarly, during assessment, questions designed to test memory and orientation may be met with extreme annoyance and an abrupt termination of the interview. It is understandable that people will not wish to expose their failings or dependence on others as they try to hold on to a conviction that 'all is well'.

Reality confrontation

Exposing a confused person to the painfulness of a present characterised by a loss of persons, places and things can result in anger and abuse as they live and know a reality of years ago. This response will be all the more vociferous and violent if carers, exhausted and exasperated, lose sensitivity and become 'brutal' in the way they convey information that 'is not true'.

Alarm

Abrupt and rapid approaches toward a vulnerable person – possibly poorly sighted, hard of hearing, as well as disoriented – especially if coming from behind or involving unexpected physical contact, can easily result in a hostile act of self-protection. Bear in mind that our normal pace is likely to be too fast for an elderly person, slowed by age and affected by poor hearing and eyesight.

Misunderstanding events

Trying to make sense of an uncertain and mysterious world can easily result in misunderstanding and inappropriate actions. For example, a disoriented man may believe the district nurse who visits his frail wife is assaulting her; a homecare worker may be regarded as an unwelcome intruder, or a woman on a long-stay ward may hold a belief that fellow patients should respect her privacy and go home. Such misunderstanding can, understandably, be responsible for aggressive actions.

Manipulation

In the beginning, when a person retains the cognitive capacity to reason and recall, aggression may be used as a means to manipulate others in order to get their own way. Without the necessary intellectual and memory abilities, this explanation is highly improbable.

Psychosis

Aggression has been linked to delusional ideation. In one study it was observed that people with dementia who experienced delusions were four times more likely to be at least mildly aggressive (Gormley *et al*, 1998). It does not appear that hallucinations are related to aggressive acts.

Attention-seeking

Even though violent behaviour and threatening gestures are uncommon, when they occur those affected are understandably watchful and ill at ease. As a result they are a powerful means of gaining attention. However, the factors we need to consider when deciding whether 'manipulation' is the reason for aggressive behaviour are also relevant to this potential explanation.

Adaptive paranoia

This example of verbal aggression is not evidence of psychosis. Blaming others is a means by which the frightening implications of a deteriorating memory are denied. Making accusations against others to explain why items cannot be found or why an arrangement was forgotten can provide external sources of blame for internally caused mistakes. As such, attempts to hide incompetence are early rather than late features of dementia, and the accusations may at first appear plausible. However, given the risk of older adult abuse and the tendency for others to disempower those with dementia, it is unwise to automatically assume that accusations of mistreatment are without substance.

Goal frustration

Aggression may be the reaction to a carer's response to confine or control the drives and desires of those with dementia. Giving instructions to stop or to act differently may provoke an aggressive gesture, as will physical restraint. A person who wanders away from the house, or is entering the rooms of others, may react with hostility when prevented from doing so. Or maybe it is when a woman tries to live her home life as she has always done, but unwittingly attempts to put cartons of milk in the oven. Physically preventing her from such hazardous conduct may result in her 'lashing out, and thrashing me with a tea towel' (the words of a desperate husband). In some people the unwillingness to comply with instructions presents as a wilful attempt to do the opposite of what is requested. Faced with unremitting refusal and frustration, carers feel they cannot do right for doing wrong. This is consistent with the 'age of negativism' observed at the beginnings of selfhood.

During self-care tasks a person may become frustrated and angry because apraxia interferes with the voluntary control of movements. The outcome is a marked impairment of daily living skills, which results in frustration and the prospect that well-meaning assistance may in turn be resisted as the person acts out their irritation. This is most likely to happen when a carer fails to appreciate the frustration felt, and instead assumes there is simply a task to be done.

Similarly, a person may experience the frustration of being unable to communicate their needs because speech is affected by expressive aphasia. Frustration-related anger can be compounded when others who are trying to piece together what is being said arrive at obscure interpretations, to the exasperation of the person who is struggling to make themselves understood. The listener's mistaken reasoning is that if what the person wished to say was simple and straightforward, the words would be produced. As this is not happening, the person must be trying to articulate a complex communication and hence their attempts to 'fill in the gaps' drift into the obscure and irrelevant.

Some researchers (eg Hamel *et al*, 1990) have raised the possibility that a person is more likely to respond aggressively when faced with frustrating situations if their pre-morbid way had always been to do so.

While this may account for a proportion of hostile incidents, on many occasions the abuse and aggressive posturing appear 'out of character'.

Impulsive over-reaction

An unexpected change of routine, a misplaced article of value, or a name that cannot be recalled may result in a poorly controlled outburst of temper, or possibly even rage, as a result of frontal-lobe brain damage.

With only a few exceptions there is great aetiological value in knowing the setting in which aggression arises. Researchers (eg, Ware *et al*, 1990; Gormley *et al*, 1998) have observed aggressive behaviour occurring most often during intimate care, when responding to instructions, or in response to the aggressive acts of others.

The aggressive outburst

Carers often describe the difficulties they experience in coping with people who behave aggressively. This is understandable, for to be the victim of a physical attack or verbal abuse is distressing. Yet, as has been revealed at length, aggressive acts rarely occur without reason. Thus prevention is always the favoured way of working. On occasions, however, acts of hostility are unexpected and inexplicable. Sometimes we let ourselves down and initiate an ambiguous, and possibly alarming, approach. In these instances we require knowledge and skill to respond appropriately, so preventing the episode from escalating out of hand.

Bryan and Maxim (1994) provide useful guidance on how to work with a person who is shouting, swearing or accusing.

- Try to stay calm.
- Do not take the insults personally.
- Back away so personal space is not infringed and maintain eye contact (but do not glare).
- Give calm reassurance that all is well.
- While speaking slowly and gently, explain why you are with them.
- If verbal abuse persists, disengage and inform them that you will return later.
- Attempt to determine the explanation for their abusive conduct, and then try again.

If carers are faced with a violent incident, the objective is to reduce the risk of injury to themselves, the person who is being aggressive and any bystanders, some of whom may be frail.

What not to do

1 Do not be confrontational.
2 Do not raise your voice.
3 Do not attempt to lead the person away or initiate any other form of physical contact, as such actions can easily be misunderstood.
4 Do not stay in their personal space (this varies from person to person, but at a time of distress a distance of about one metre is a useful estimate).
5 Do not corner the person, as this will heighten feelings of threat and alarm.
6 Do not crowd them by calling for assistance.
7 Do not tease or ridicule.
8 Do not attempt to use restraints.
9 Do not show fear, alarm or anxiety as this may not only serve to encourage the violent act, but also may cause agitation by demonstrating that it is not only they who are unable to cope, but you as well.

Recommended practice

If we are to feel confident in our ability to cope with violent behaviour, we need to know what is expected of us at such times. The following responses – not all of which will be relevant in every aggressive episode – are essential if we are to de-escalate violent situations:

1 By staying calm you demonstrate you are in control.
2 Respect their personal space. This serves to reduce threat and enables carers to maintain a safe distance. Rather than facing the person directly, stand at an angle of 45 degrees. Ensure there are no items that can be reached that are likely to injure.
3 Try to convey reassurance by tone of voice, but also be firm so boundaries of acceptable behaviour are appreciated. This is known as 'limit setting'.

4 If appropriate, and if possible, ask or direct other people to draw back and not to interfere. Be concerned for those who are vulnerable.

5 Encourage them to talk rather than act out their anger. Engage eye contact and practise skills of active listening (Stokes, 2000).

6 Ask the person what is troubling them. Try to identify why they are so angry. Voice tone should remain constant and not reflect irritation or tension.

7 Listen to what they say. Be accepting, not rejecting. Acknowledge their feelings; do not embark on correction and justification. Seek points of similarity rather than difference. Try to agree to something, thus building the first small bond of cooperation. Deal with the 'here and now', rather than issues from the past.

8 Try to divert their attention if they remain angry. Give them the psychological room to move from their aroused state. Offer a way out by providing alternatives to the behaviour. Keep options simple.

The objective of these actions is to defuse the situation. It is to be hoped that an empathic, responsive, but firm reaction will enable the person to calm down. At this point, someone else – if possible their keyworker, for they know them best – should talk to them. If they will accompany that person, this could happen somewhere quiet, away from the site of the incident. A gentle conversation in a tranquil area will be a 'holding' response to an upsetting experience (see Kitwood, 1996).

The carer involved in the aggressive episode should be given the opportunity to talk through what happened with colleagues. There is no blaming, but a wish to learn from the episode, such as how well did we respond to the person's anger, and what are the underlying needs we must try to meet in order to prevent a similar episode in the future?

The victim who is at serious risk
If the person has lost control and is in danger of injuring themselves, or if they are attacking somebody else who is vulnerable, caregivers need to respond effectively:

• No more than two carers are needed to intervene.
• Approach from the front, with speed but not haste.

- They should not be wearing anything visible that could be potentially harmful if it were to be grabbed.
- They need to speak in a calm but matter-of-fact manner, requesting the person to stop or let go.
- A commentary should be provided to inform the person what is happening and what the carers' intentions are.
- If the assault continues, as a last resort and using minimal force, the carers should take hold of each arm and disengage the person from the victim. No other physical contact is necessary. During this action the talking continues, reassuring the person and their victim that all will soon be well.
- Once the two are separated, the victim can be comforted by one of the carers.
- The other carer breaks away from the aggressor, respects their personal space, and talks to them in accordance with the guidelines for responding to a violent episode.

By following these recommendations on how to communicate with a person who is aggressive, and possibly violent, carers can avoid a traumatic confrontation at a time when everybody involved is feeling at their most vulnerable.

The need to break away
Even though such situations are few and far between, if a carer is at risk from assault and there is no hope of de-escalation, only legitimate and reasonable force necessary for defence can be employed to break away.

Reasonable force is force that is no more than is necessary to accomplish disengagement, and must be in proportion to the harm which is threatened.

Actions in accordance with self-defence are, however, only legitimate when there has been *no prior opportunity to retreat and walk away*. To choose to remain is to commit an assault.

Abuse
While not being the true focus of this chapter, we learnt in Chapter 8 of Mr Bryan, a man who acted out a frustration-related assault against a

woman with severe dementia (pp85–7). Carers may also intentionally or unwittingly commit acts of physical abuse, possibly when caring for an abusive or resistive relative or client. Cooney and Howard (1995) suggest that 'Elderly people with dementia living with a carer are at a significantly higher risk of abuse than the general population over 65.' Another study reported that nearly 12 per cent of carers had physically abused their relative (Coyne *et al*, 1993). Without doubt most people care with compassion and devotion. A few, however, at times of exasperation, having been driven to their wits end, lose control and find their tolerance eclipsed by hostility and anger. Similarly, professional carers may act harshly when provoked, or they may engage in ill-advised restraint.

So when we next hear of a person who wanders away from their home; calls out 'help me', or is said to be resistive, could it be possible they are trying to leave an abusive setting, communicating their experience of abuse, or attempting to push away a perpetrator? As these signs are more likely to be seen as 'symptoms of disease', the vulnerability of people with dementia cannot be exaggerated.

References

Bryan K & Maxim J, 1994, 'How Not To Give As Good As You Get', *Journal of Dementia Care* 2, pp25–7.

Cooney C & Howard R, 1995, 'Abuse of Patients with Dementia by Carers – Out of Sight But Not Out of Mind', *International Journal of Geriatric Psychiatry* 10, pp735–41.

Coyne A, Reichman W & Berbig L, 1993, 'The Relationship between Dementia and Elder Abuse', *American Journal of Psychiatry* 146, pp184–97.

Dean R, Briggs K & Lindesey J, 1993, 'The Domus Philosophy: A Prospective Evaluation of Two Residential Units for the Elderly Mentally Ill', *International Journal of Geriatric Psychiatry* 9, pp807–17.

Gormley N, Rizwan MR & Lovestone S, 1998, 'Clinical Predictors of Aggressive Behaviour in Alzheimer's Disease', *International Journal of Geriatric Psychiatry* 13, pp109–15.

Hamel M, Gold DP, Andres D, Reis M, Dastoor D, Graver H & Bergman H, 1990, 'Prediction and Consequences of Aggressive Behaviour by Community Based Dementia Patients', *The Gerontologist* 30, pp206–11.

Hope RA, Keane J, Fairburn C, McShane R & Jacoby R, 1997, 'Behaviour Changes in Dementia II: Are There Behavioural Syndromes?', *International Journal of Geriatric Psychiatry* 5, pp239–45.

Inness A, 1998, 'Behind Labels: What Makes Behaviour Difficult?', *Journal of Dementia Care* 6(5), pp22–5.

Kitwood T, 1996, 'A Dialectical Framework for Dementia', in Woods RT (ed), *Handbook of the Clinical Psychology of Ageing*, John Wiley, Chichester.

Patel V & Hope RA, 1992, 'Aggressive Behaviour in a Hospitalised Psychogeriatric Population', *Acta Psychiatrica, Scandinavica* 85, pp131–5.

Shah AK, 1991, 'Low Levels of Violence on a Psychogeriatric Ward', *Geriatric Medicine* 21, p27.

Shah AK, 1992, 'Violence and Psychogeriatric Inpatients', *International Journal of Geriatric Psychiatry* 7, pp39–44.

Stokes G, 2000, *Challenging Behaviour in Dementia*, Speechmark Publishing/Winslow Press, Bicester.

Ware CJG, Fairburn CG & Hope RA, 1990, 'A Community-Based Study of Aggressive Behaviour in Dementia', *International Journal of Geriatric Psychiatry* 5, pp337–42.

CHAPTER 14

Wandering: We Walk, They Wander!

Graham Stokes

'WANDERING IS OFTEN ONE OF THE FIRST symptoms that gets an individual living in the community into trouble, or puts him or her in danger' (Burnside, 1980). Rabins *et al* (1982) reported that 40 per cent of family carers found wandering to be a troublesome problem. For those carers who find the need to provide constant supervision stressful, the strain can promote a range of coping strategies as extreme as physical restraints, chemical control (medication and alcohol) and 'aggression' (Dodds, 1994). Yet, what is meant by wandering?

Most reports of the prevalence of wandering in dementia are flawed by the lack of both a clear definition of the behaviour and a reliable method of assessment. As a result, it is possibly the most misused and abused descriptive label employed in the area of challenging behaviour.

Operational definition

Behavioural definition
Wandering is a single-minded determination to walk that is unresponsive to persuasion:
a) With no or only superficial awareness for personal safety (eg, an inability to return, or impaired recognition of hazard)
b) With no apparent regard for others (eg, in terms of time of day, duration, frequency or privacy)

c) With no regard for personal welfare (thereby disrupting the essential behaviours of eating, sleeping and resting).

The behavioural definition distinguishes between wandering with risk (a) and wandering as nuisance (b), as well as interpreting walking as wandering if the behaviour is 'to excess' (c), even though there is no risk or disturbance to others. The final element of the definition accommodates the finding that, following entry to a secure environment to live alongside others who rarely, if ever, respond, a person's 'abnormal walking' is relegated to the status of an unacknowledged behaviour, for their actions are less likely to trigger the threshold of concern. The absence of risk or nuisance should not, however, generate complacency or inertia to the point where the pursuit of understanding and resolution is deemed unnecessary.

Without this definition, the behavioural characteristics listed below (some of which are common to those established in the community survey of Hope and Fairburn, 1990) may attract the label of 'wandering' as soon as a person with dementia walks. The restrictions on activity that may follow can in turn result in a sedentary lifestyle and actions that may even contravene basic human rights (Mayer & Darby, 1991). Without doubt, the equation to avoid is that if wandering equals walking, then walking must equal wandering (see Figure 14.1).

Behavioural characteristics
The following behavioural characteristics describe activities that can take place outside or indoors, or result in an attempt to go outside. It is undeniable, however, that the type and location of the behaviour will influence whether the actions are judged to be evidence of wandering or not (Albert, 1992; Sayer, 1994).

• Pottering with purpose (busying themselves)
• Following behaviour (walking behind or hovering around others)
• Apparently aimless walking
• Pacing/restless movement
• Comfortable remnants (pursuing tasks from the past)

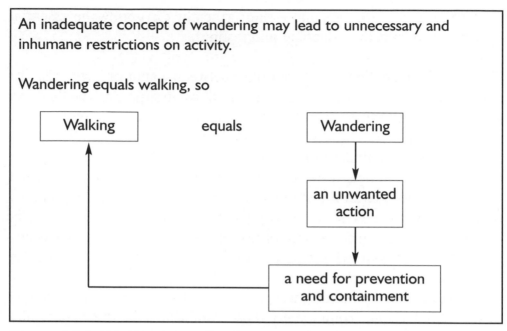

An inadequate concept of wandering may lead to unnecessary and inhumane restrictions on activity.

Wandering equals walking, so

Walking   equals   Wandering

an unwanted action

a need for prevention and containment

Figure 14.1 *Wandering or walking?*

- Trailing/tracking a significant other (clinging to a carer)
- Searching for their past (going home, going to work or seeking children)
- Attachment behaviour (when apart, seeking the proximity of a person or place that represents security)
- Over-appropriate functional or comfortable behaviour (eg, excessive frequency)
- Exit behaviour (persistent efforts to 'get out')
- Place disorientation (getting lost within a building)
- Walking with risk in pursuit of an appropriate goal
- Appropriate functional or comfortable behaviours at an inappropriate time.

Wandering – why might it be happening?

Appreciating that we all, regardless of intellectual status, need to walk, if a person's behaviour does fall within the operational definition of wandering there is no single explanation to account for the behaviour. Wandering, as with most challenging behaviours, does not constitute a coherent syndrome. Instead there are different kinds of wandering, each of which has its own explanation. If we refer to the behavioural characteristics, a person who 'potters with purpose' is unlikely to indulge in 'exit behaviour' or 'trailing and tracking', for each are the behavioural consequences of different motivations. Unless needs change, other wandering 'characteristics' are unlikely to appear, and rarely will we observe simultaneous expression unless the actions share a common motivational bond.

Separation anxiety

When in the company of another whose presence provides reassurance and peace of mind, all is relatively well. Unfortunately, as that person lives their life, they move around the house, or go out. The fragmentation of experience means that there is no recollection of where they have gone, how long they have been away, or any message to the effect that they will return. They are just absent. Separation anxiety motivates those with dementia to cling to this other person ('trailing and tracking'), or if the person with dementia is removed to another setting in order to give their family respite from the suffocating pressure of being 'trailed', they will attempt to leave so they may seek the whereabouts of those significant others ('attachment behaviour').

Confusion

A person with dementia may become confused in an attempt to find somebody who or something that is unobtainable because it resides in their past. Searching for young children; going home and seeking deceased loved ones, usually parents or a spouse, are commonly observed. Their determination to 'search for their past' is borne out of conviction and invariably does not benefit from reality orientation. To us their walking is directed towards an inappropriate goal, but that is not how it is to them.

Habits of a lifetime

People with dementia may indulge in actions that are confused continuations of what they once did. These 'comfortable remnants' are now inappropriate to the new context – for example, walking around at night 'securing' the residential unit before going to bed. The behaviours may be related to parenting, occupation or home life.

Living life
As they carry out the practical tasks of daily life and pursue comfortable behaviours, the pursuit of these in appropriate goals may be intrusive. Memory deficits, time disorientation and poor judgement result in the person becoming a nuisance if the task is carried out with inappropriate frequency (for example, watering houseplants throughout the day; visiting the post office hour after hour; checking to see if the front door is closed), or they may cause concern if they are no longer able to appreciate danger or know that they will become lost. The challenge to others may be that the motivation is inappropriate at the time chosen ('appropriate goal, inappropriate time'). Examples would be going to the shops when they are closed; leaving to visit relatives in the early hours of the morning, or attempting to walk in the garden during the hours of darkness. This explanation integrates the effects of cognitive impairment with the knowledge of a person's uniqueness and their subjective appreciation of a life to be lived.

Physical discomfort
As walking can ease discomfort, and even distract us from our suffering, a person with dementia may start to walk around. Unable to articulate a reason for their excessive activity, we see 'apparently aimless' or 'restless' movement.

Coping with stress
To pace is a stress response (as in 'the caged animal' or 'the expectant father'). Some people go for a walk when they are troubled. These are further explanations for 'restless pacing'.

Failure of navigation
An inability to store new experiences or recall previously learned information will result in a person becoming lost within a building as they try to locate, for example, their bedroom or the toilet ('place disorientation').

Boredom

Inactivity motivates a person with dementia 'to do'. As they walk around busying themselves their actions are purposeful, even though the observed actions may be bizarre – for example, gathering, moving furniture, or manipulating objects. While their wandering may be a nuisance to us, 'pottering with purpose' is a source of contentment. If their 'pottering' is reminiscent of known patterns of behaving, then it is categorised as a 'comfortable behaviour', possibly an historical remnant.

Loneliness

The person with dementia who lives alone may leave their home to find companionship. The motivation is not inappropriate; the challenge is that they do not appreciate the risks involved ('walking with risk toward an appropriate goal'), or the appropriate purpose is repeated to excess ('over-appropriate behaviour'). In communal settings, it is not that they are isolated, but 'being alone in a crowd' motivates them to walk around in an effort to find a friendly face to be with. This may result in 'following behaviour'.

Curiosity

A person may wander as they search for meaning and answers. We observe 'apparently aimless walking', 'exit behaviour', or 'place disorientation'.

Fear

In an unfamiliar place or faced with the strangeness of others, those with dementia may be so frightened they are desperate to leave ('exit behaviour'). Alternatively, they may roam around unsuccessfully seeking sanctuary. Disorientation may add to their fear.

Avoidance behaviour

A person who is unable to voice their complaints may seek to escape from unpleasant environmental 'noise'. Sitting by the meaningless stimulation of a television; having to endure age-inappropriate background music, or the calling out of others can understandably result in them trying to get out and becoming lost, or apparently walking without purpose once the motivation to walk has been forgotten.

Perseveration

Frontal-lobe damage may result in walking to excess for no reason. Perseveration means that a person's actions are not under voluntary control. Malcolm, a 50-year-old man with probable Pick's disease, does very little other than walk continuously around his home. He has a set route that he follows; through the lounge, along the hall, through the kitchen and back into the lounge. Having completed his circuit many times, he will sit for a few moments before getting up and starting again.

Mirroring

We observe certain residents in care who will leave their chairs to follow another person, for no other reason than that person started to walk. 'Mirroring' results in 'following behaviour' and is possibly motivated by the security found in the 'herd instinct'. A person, insecure and not knowing, sees another 'leaving' and follows because by going elsewhere that person is 'felt' to be dominant and knowing.

Spatial agnosia

Spatial agnosia will make it so difficult for a person to find their way around, even in buildings known well, that they will end up lost as they try to identify 'landmarks' that make sense.

Sundowning

Agitated, purposeless wandering or determined exit behaviour may occur at the end of the day. Often known as 'sundowning', this may be the consequence of cellular destruction producing diurnal rhythm disturbance (see Stokes, 2000). However, it may have psychological roots. From our earliest years we are accustomed to departing as the day ends. We went home from school, we go home from work. Triggered by both internal and external cues, the person with dementia may start to move around in early evening for no apparent reason.

Fragmentation of experience

A person may get up with a task or plan in mind, but then forget what they had intended to do, ending up wandering aimlessly with no apparent motive.

Given the variety of reasons that motivate us to walk, it is hardly surprising that the same richness of motivation underpins a tendency to wander. No longer can it be said that a person with dementia wanders *because* they have dementia.

Wandering – ways to cope

It is not always possible to resolve the challenge of wandering. At such times the question that typifies the old culture of care can be resurrected, 'how are we going to manage …'? If wandering cannot be resolved, this is a legitimate question. In the absence of solution, psychological and practical strategies, some more effective than others, may enable us to manage better.

The provision of sensible security precautions helps reduce unnecessary risk and allows both family and professional carers to know that a crisis is less likely to occur. In the pursuit of peace of mind, I am not advocating a policy of protective custody, just sensible precautions to generate confidence among carers that the person is not exposed to undue and disproportionate risk.

Personal information

Providing information such as name, address and telephone number on a card placed in a wallet, purse or pocket, or even on a label stitched inside the jacket or overcoat, may aid a speedy return home if someone gets lost. It is important, however, that the information is carried in a way that does not signpost the person as an individual at risk.

Alarms

Alarms can be employed when professional caregivers have limited time to be watchful of the exits. Alarms can be triggered whenever a secured door is opened. Where such a system would be too intrusive, electronic tagging has been advocated. Triggered by a small tag fitted into the clothing of a person, the doors are open to all except those who are 'tagged'. However, there are certain issues and questions that need to be addressed when the use of electronic tagging is being considered (see Table 14.1).

The most significant reservation does not, however, relate to issues of implementation, but pertains to the ethical issue of 'tagging' someone.

Table 14.1 *Implications of electronic tagging*

Issue	Questions
The alarm must be unobtrusive so as not to distress either the person who is leaving, or others in care.	Will there be sufficient staff to monitor a discreet alarm that may only be heard in the exit area or, if connected to a master console, in the office? If not, are mobile receivers available?
The electronic tag needs to be attached to clothing.	It is possible that the article of clothing could be removed by the person, thereby overcoming the alarm system. A danger is that 'tagging' can breed a false sense of security among staff.
A 'triggered' alarm system enables doors to be left 'open'.	A situation could arise wherein a 'tagged' person could lead out another resident with dementia who may remain outside unobserved and at risk.

Because of the potentially fatal consequences, getting lost outside the home is one of the most worrying developments for carers. Tagging devices offer a solution, as do electronic transmitters that enable a person to be tracked down if they are missing.

While Marshall (1995) argues that technology 'is the shape of the future whether we like it or not', she accepts that we 'have to find a balance between the duty of care and freedom of choice'. The technology may benefit carers, but it may also be associated with degrading and dehumanising treatment, that is not in the 'best interest' of the person (see Stokes, 2001).

McShane *et al* (1994) propose that in the right circumstances tagging devices are desirable. If by leaving a building a person would be harmed (eg, knocked down by a car), as well as placing others at risk (eg, the driver involved in the accident), 'a degree of restriction of freedom is a price worth paying for the safety of the person and others.' McShane *et al* (1994) propose a similar argument for tracking devices – 'if it is ethically proper to search for them, surely it would be proper to do so with the help of a tracking device.' It can even be argued that the use of this technology might enhance liberty by enabling a less restrictive form of care.

There is much to commend the view that a considered application of surveillance technology benefits the person with dementia, yet as Marshall (1995) declares, the need for safeguards to avoid abuse is equally compelling.

These would include:

- Operational definition of the 'problem'
- A record of the efforts made to resolve the behaviour
- Discussions with relatives and the appointment of an advocate
- A decision to be made on the use of technology to 'manage' the behaviour
- Documentation to record the behaviour and wellbeing of the person
- Specified time for review and who will be involved;

A simple alarm system that can be installed at the main entrance of a day centre or residential home is to connect the opening of the front door to the doorbell. Whenever the door is opened the bell sounds. Such a device is both unobtrusive and 'normal', and can be used easily within a person's own home. If the system is used at a day centre or in a continuing care setting where, for example, the main entrance is in constant use, the use of a digital code can prevent the bell ringing. The code is displayed by the door, and if it is punched in prior to the door being opened, the bell will not sound. As a person with dementia is unlikely to master the procedure (although those with frontal-lobe dementia may well be able to), when the bell sounds carers are alerted.

The introduction of a 'doorbell alarm' had an unexpected, albeit beneficial outcome in the case of a man who persistently attempted to leave a day centre to go home – home being Belfast, a journey of more than 300 miles! On opening the front door, the bell rang. He would stop, look outside, see nobody there, scowl and then, muttering to himself, step back inside and close the door!

Marshall (1995) also described 'passive alarms', which can be placed under a mat beside the side of a bed or by interior doors to alert carers that a person is walking around the home. They are triggered when someone steps on them.

Locks

The locking of doors is not to be encouraged in continuing care establishments, but if the person with dementia lives at home the security of the front door does not constitute an infringement of personal liberty. If a carer is to be free of the need to mount a constant watch and have a sound night's sleep without worrying about whether a partner has slipped out of the house under the cover of darkness, locking the front door is an essential measure.

As people with dementia have difficulty in storing fresh information and learning new ways, a new lock on the door can be a significant barrier to leaving the house. The more complex the lock, the less likely it is that the problem will be solved. Locating a lock in an unfamiliar position, such as at the top or bottom of the front door, will make the opening of the door an even more complicated task. This is an alternative to a lock that is difficult to operate.

A safety measure used in care settings is to employ 'baffle handles' that need to be pulled simultaneously in opposite directions. These difficult-to-operate handles help to prevent the possible dangers of wandering, while providing maximum opportunity for physical activity within a designated area. Similarly, the use of digital locks that can puzzle the more able person with dementia who can overcome the 'baffle' system can be effective. Access to the establishment or unit can be 'open', but to leave the facility requires input of the digital code. Again, this can be displayed by the door for the benefit of visitors.

As with tagging and tracking technology, the introduction of locks and baffle systems raises concerns over individual liberty. Yet it can again be argued that such security initiatives can lead to a more relaxed, less repressive, care regime. It is not the security of the exits that should warrant greatest debate, but what is happening behind the doors that are now secured. Such a policy encourages freedom of movement within the building rather than placing limitations on walking; it enables one-to-one activities as carers do not have to group people together in order to exercise a watchful eye, and it avoids the dedication of scarce staff time to surveillance duties by the main exit.

Secured doors can be integral to effective dementia care, but they should be employed judiciously; not be seen as an alternative to staff, and at all times the use of locks or similar barriers must be compatible with the requirements laid down by fire and safety regulations. The environment must ensure safety, but it cannot be the overriding theme of design.

Perimeter boundaries

Securing the external perimeter can act as a fail-safe response, or possibly an alternative to baffling or locking doors. If it is safe for someone to walk outside then restrictions on leaving a building have low priority.

While secure perimeters conjure up visions of high fences and imposing gates, this is far removed from what can be achieved with creative thought.

At home, a bolt on the far side of the gate, best placed at the base, can be an insurmountable barrier.

In continuing care establishments, as an alternative to fences, garden landscaping can deter people from leaving. People rarely walk across grass, let alone trample through flower beds, so a design that incorporates circular paths that meander through oases of colour and interest, raised flower beds, rose bushes with attractive trellis work behind and hedges can disguise the objective of establishing perimeter security.

Internal design

Some people have noted the benefits of simple environmental changes. 'Wandering circuits' have been proposed (eg, Beck & Shue, 1994), while others have suggested that floor patterns, especially horizontal stripes before an exit door (Hewawasum, 1996) may reduce attempts to leave a home. Disguising a door by painting it the same colour as the adjacent walls will reduce its interest value and diminish the likelihood that it will be noticed. Doors can be disguised by attractive and creative wall coverings, such as book shelves reminiscent of a library.

At night a curtain or blind may be an effective means of disguise (eg, Dickinson *et al*, 1995). As this is not a constant environmental feature, the association between door and curtain is unlikely to be established. This is unlikely to work if the person lives at home, for it is overlearned knowledge that the front door is located at the end of a hallway.

Attaching a full-length mirror to internal doors will make recognition difficult (eg, Mayer & Darby, 1991). However, this design initiative needs to be balanced against the possibility of heightened disorientation, agitation and the risk of injury if the mirror is not properly secured.

All building and design adaptations to manage the risks and nuisance of wandering must avoid a sense of confinement. We are attempting to create a safe environment, not one that is unduly restrictive and thus a source of frustration. A distressing feature of dementia care is to see people banging on windows, persistently pulling at door handles, or forlornly standing at a gate they cannot open. Their quality of life cannot be ignored just because they are no longer a cause for concern. 'It may be better to accept a small degree of risk than to hem a person in completely ...' (Kitwood & Bredin, 1992). This may sometimes conflict with the caution of relatives. Their worries cannot be dismissed. We need to talk about the unacceptability of physical and pharmacological restraint, and the need to provide a secure but caring environment, with due regard for rights, as well as the potential for risk.

Psychosocial intervention

When somebody leaves a building, if it is possible accompany them. Nothing more is required. Just walk with them for a while. If they take your arm their wandering now becomes a stroll. If this approach is not feasible, and often this will be so, the following intervention involving two staff members can often work:

- Let the person walk away from the building for several moments (the length of time will be influenced by the range of safe distance).
- The first carer approaches the person and walks alongside them for a minute or so. No attempt is made to encourage them to return, unless the person wishes to do so. Striking up a conversation makes it a social happening.
- The second carer now approaches and asks both of them to return. If the person 'wandering' does not agree, the first carer says they will return shortly. The second carer goes back.

- Several moments later, the first carer suggests they both return. It is surprising how often the strategy works. The explanations for the method's effectiveness are likely to include:
  - a trusting bond has been established ('holding')
  - with the passage of time, the motivation for leaving has been forgotten
  - the person may already be getting tired or cold
  - what faces them is unknown; what is behind is felt as known, and so it feels safer to return than to venture forth.

These psychosocial measures help prevent confrontation and need to 'be weighed against the alternatives, which are often psychoactive medication used for restraint' (Moniz-Cook, 1998).

References

Albert SM, 1992, 'The Nature of Wandering in Dementia: a Guttman Scaling Analysis of an Empirical Classifaction Scheme', *International Journal of Geriatric Psychiatry* 7, pp783–7.

Beck CK & Shue VM, 1994, 'Interventions for Treating Disruptive Behaviour in Demented Elderly People', *Nursing Clinics of North America* 29, pp143–55.

Burnside IM, 1980, *Nursing Care of the Aged,* 2nd edn, McGraw-Hill, New York.

Dickinson J, McLain-Kark & Marshall-Baker J, 1995, 'The Effects of Visual Barriers on Existing Behaviour in a Dementia Care Unit', *The Gerontologist* 35, pp126–30.

Dodds P, 1994, 'Wandering: A Short Report on Coping Strategies Adopted by Informal Carers', *International Journal of Geriatric Psychiatry* 9, pp751–6.

Hewawasum L, 1996, 'Floor Patterns Limit Wandering of People with Alzheimer's', *Nursing Times* 92(23), pp41–4.

Hope RA & Fairburn CG, 1990, 'The Nature of Wandering in Dementia: a community based study', *International Journal of Geriatric Psychiatry* 5, pp239–45.

Kitwood T & Bredin K, 1992, *Person to Person,* Gale Centre Publications, Loughton.

Marshall M, 1995, 'Technology is the Shape of the Future', *Journal of Dementia Care* 3(3), pp12–14.

Mayer R & Darby SJ, 1991, 'Does a Mirror Deter Wandering in Demented Older People?', *International Journal of Geriatric Psychiatry* 6, pp607–9.

McShane R, Hope T & Wilkinson J, 1994, 'Tracking Patients Who Wander: Ethics and Technology', *The Lancet* 343, p1274.

Moniz-Cook E, 1998, 'Psychosocial Approaches to "Challenging Behaviour" in Care Homes', *Journal of Dementia Care* 6(5), pp33–8.

Rabins PV, Mace HL & Lucas MJ, 1982, 'The Impact of Dementia on the Family', *Journal of the American Medical Association* 248, pp333–5.

Sayer RJ, 1994, 'The Management of Wandering in Nursing and Residential Homes: is there a role for occupational therapy?', unpublished report, School of Health and Social Sciences, Coventry University.

Stokes G, 2000, *Challenging Behaviour in Dementia*, Speechmark Publishing/Winslow Press, Bicester.

Stokes G, 2001, 'Difficult Decisions: What Are a Person's 'Best Interests?'', *Journal of Dementia Care* 9, pp25–8.

CHAPTER 15

Confusion

Graham Stokes

THE ESSENCE OF MOST PEOPLE'S understanding of dementia is that the person is confused. Yet the term 'confusion' encompasses a vast range of behaviours, which only share in common the observation that others find them puzzling and inappropriate. As such, usage in itself can be confusing. People are said to be confused if they are restless, uncooperative, forgetful or disoriented.

To bring precision to the concept, confusion can be distinguished from actions that implicate error (eg, placing objects in the 'wrong' place); poor judgement (eg, putting flammable items on the cooker or drinking from the washing-up bowl); disorientation (eg, lost and bewildered), and hallucinations and delusions typical of psychosis. As such, the following behavioural definition excludes mistake, misjudgement, 'not knowing' and psychotic phenomena. Alternative definitions are not wrong, but have simply adopted a different psycho-behavioural framework.

Behavioural definition
Confusion is the reporting of information or living of experience that represents a reality discordant to our own.

Behavioural characteristics
• Claiming deceased parents or partners are alive
• Demanding to go to work

- Wanting to find or care for their young children
- Leaving home to go 'home'
- Talking to strangers or professional carers as if they are 'loved ones'
- Knowing partners to be parents, and adult children to be partners
- Acting inappropriate to context (eg, knowing themselves to be at work when they are in day-care).

The challenge of confusion

In some ways confusion presents us with our greatest challenge. How do we bring peace of mind to a person who knows her children are lost, or their mother is waiting for them at home? How do we meet their needs? We cannot; all we can do is to alleviate their torment.

Reality orientation

We have seen that RO has a role to play in ameliorating disorientation (see Chapter 9). Yet is it a therapeutic option to employ when working with the needs of those who are confused? Can we reduce confusion by correcting confused speech and challenging confused actions? Probably not. When attempting to help a confused person, the frustration of caregivers is not that they do not learn, as is the case with disorientation, but that they do not believe. When carers are faced with a person's desperate pleading for partners, parents or children, our efforts to inform, possibly reassure, degenerate into reality confrontation. They simply will not accept our reality. 'It seems so confrontational and possibly distressing to attempt to orientate them to our current reality' (Woods, 1994). This turn of events is not surprising, for we now appreciate that their reality is a world of conviction, not belief. If our reality is not amenable to correction then how can theirs be?

Yet is confrontation inevitable? The answer is no. It is often observed that as carers become exasperated they apply RO in an insensitive and, on occasions, brutal manner. They practise on a cognitive level, focusing on facts and logic.

On these occasions the approach is misapplied. There has been a disregard for feelings and a loss of regard for the person. There is preoccupation with cognitive deficits and an objectification of the individual. We must learn that showing respect for the individual and demonstrating empathy for their feeling experience take 'primacy over any approach or technique' (Woods, 1994). Caregivers need to appreciate the need for wellbeing and then decide when, how or even if they should be presented with reality. Yet what if our judgement is that RO, even when communicated with humanity will not only fail to progress awareness, but is likely to cause distress, what are we to do?

Time-shift

Holden (1990) advocates a hybrid of RO and distraction known as 'time-shift' when communicating with a person who steadfastly holds on to their reality. If they demand to go home to be with their mother, it may be appropriate to say, 'It must have been nice when your mother *was* at home with you. What *was* she like?' The past tense is used with care, acknowledging their feelings and yet correcting the time perspective. In due course, the objective of the communication is to bring the person into present reality by saying 'You must miss her very much.' If the final step of reality awareness is likely to produce trauma, I have found that simply reminiscing, and hence achieving an accurate 'time-shift', may be rewarding and may also reduce the motivation to 'search'.

Holden (1990) acknowledges that the approach 'might be resented'. The technique is a welcome addition to our therapeutic armoury, but the prospect of avoiding confrontation must be tempered with realism, if not caution.

Collusion

When we agree with a person's perception of reality, that is collusion.

- 'At times he asks the staff when his mother is going to visit next. Some staff members tell him that his mother will be visiting later in the day.'
- '... the patient has refused to eat while she insists on knowing whether her mother fixed the meal. Staff have found that she will only eat if told that her mother did indeed prepare the food.' (Dietch *et al*, 1989)
- 'She is desperate to know where her 'boys are'. We tell her they are fine, playing next door in her neighbour's garden'.

Collusion has a role to play in dementia care, but it is a psychological response of last resort when working with confusion. The approach may reassure or soothe a person who is distressed when we know, for example that RO would precipitate an extreme reaction, or distraction would be ineffective. Unfortunately, we often see collusion employed as a general way of relating to a person who is confused. It is a means by which carers can extricate themselves from challenging interactions by simply agreeing with demands or requests, knowing full well their words will be forgotten within moments: 'I must go home. Take me home.' 'I can't at the moment, I'm busy. But I'll be back in a minute, and you can go then'.

The carer can move on and the confused person is placated. But look how little time has been devoted to meaningful communication. The relationship is founded on deceit and deception. If we truly hold the belief that a person with dementia is as we are, then this is a malignant interpersonal response. When all else fails, we may resort to collusion, but malign agreement should not be a characteristic of dementia care, the motivation for which is our need for a 'quieter life', while the confused person's social experience is affected by 'treachery' (Kitwood, 1990).

Validation

While RO is not a therapy aimed at uncovering, understanding and reflecting feelings (Stokes & Goudie, 1990), validation therapy (VT) (Feil, 1992) very much is.

VT disputes the need to orientate and argues that we accept 'whatever reality they are in, in order to ease distress and restore self-worth' (Morton & Bleathman, 1991). It does not concern itself with factual errors, but acknowledges that the feelings are true and these are the material for therapeutic intervention. A woman knows her children to be young and missing; we know them as adults who are safe and well. She is objectively wrong, but subjectively there is no right or wrong. This is her unquestioning experience and her feelings are real. The acceptance of the reality and 'personal truth' of another's experience is known as validation (Kitwood, 1996). It is at this point we need to distinguish validation from VT.

Morton (see Chapter 16) expresses unease with the theory of VT. It is seen as incoherent and unconvincing (Morton & Bleathman, 1995), offering little to our understanding of dementia (Goudie & Stokes, 1989). Despite, rather than because of, VT's theoretical aspirations, Feil's methods of working have enabled us to appreciate the benefits of validation when practised with confused older people. The focus of interaction is the other person's subjective experiences. If a person with dementia is wanting to go home to their mother, we do not correct or collude, but instead we try to get a sense of the emotion that is coming across with the words and empathise with their feelings of, say, worry and anxiety.

We present with calm reassurance. I find it is often best not to mention their confused demands and pleadings, but instead, to focus on the feeling tone. It is this that we reflect and explore, and as we do so their failing memory becomes our ally. The initial motivation for their distress slowly fades, to be replaced by the quality of the therapeutic interaction. Where there was once isolation and panic, that person now finds themselves relating to somebody who smiles, whose manner is gentle and respectful, whose tolerance affirms their worth, and who looks with unfrightened eyes at elements of which they are fearful (Rogers, 1980).

Ill-being is replaced by relative wellbeing and the episode becomes a 'holding' experience. This rarely happens with RO. Even though contemporary RO values the person and recognises their capacity for wellbeing, during discourse even gentle attempts to correct act as prompts, reminding the person of the source of their fears and frustrations. As a result, wellbeing is compromised as their 'confused' motivations remain accessible to awareness. Validation is more likely to achieve therapeutic gains because their 'error' is allowed to wither on the vine as our non-corrective responses concentrate instead on the expression and sharing of emotions. These emotions will be positively affected by the experience of validation.

Validation does not ensure success. It most definitely does not constitute a remedy to be used at all times with all people. Nor is it meant to replace or compete with other methods of working with confusion. It is an empathic psychosocial intervention that helps us get closer to the experience of those whose reality is very different from our own, and for whom there is no true resolution.

References

Dietch JT, Hewett LJ & Jones S, 1989, 'Adverse Effects of Reality Orientation', *Journal of the American Geriatric Society* 37, pp974–6.

Feil N, 1992, *Validation: The Feil Method,* Feil Productions, Cleveland.

Goudie F & Stokes G, 1989, 'Understanding Confusion', *Nursing Times* 85(39), pp35–7.

Holden UP, 1990, 'Reality Orientation in the 1990s', Stokes G & Goudie F (eds), *Working with Dementia*, Speechmark Publishing/Winslow Press, Bicester.

Kitwood T, 1990, 'The Dialectics of Dementia: With Particular Reference to Alzheimer's Disease', *Ageing and Society* 10, pp177–96.

Kitwood T, 1996, 'A Dialectical Framework for Dementia', in Woods RT (ed), *Handbook of the Clinical Psychology of Ageing,* John Wiley, Chichester.

Morton I & Bleathman C, 1991, 'The Effectiveness of Validation Therapy in Dementia – A Pilot Study', *International Journal of Geriatric Psychiatry* 6, pp327–30.

Morton I & Bleathman C, 1995, 'The Roots and Growth of Person-Centred Care', *Journal of Dementia Care* 3, pp 22–5.

Rogers CR, 1980, *A Way of Being,* Houghton Mifflin, Boston.

Stokes G & Goudie F, 1990, 'Confused Elderly People', in Stokes G & Goudie F (eds), *Working with Dementia*, Speechmark Publishing/Winslow Press, Bicester.

Woods RT, 1994, 'Reality Orientation', *Journal of Dementia Care* 2(2), pp 24–5.

PART 5

THERAPEUTIC INTERVENTIONS AND FAMILY SUPPORT

CHAPTER 16

Building Therapeutic Relationships with People who have Dementia

Ian Morton

THE CLOSING YEARS OF THE TWENTIETH CENTURY bore witness to the beginnings of a major change in the way that dementia care is both conceptualised and delivered. A new set of priorities emerged as caregivers became increasingly conscious of the need to address the emotional and relationship needs of people with dementia. If such needs were to be met, then the search for guidance about how caregivers might best promote the wellbeing of people with dementia had to be widened. It had to move beyond the preoccupation with the cognitive deficits that accompany dementia – an approach that resulted in the widespread use of Reality Orientation (RO) whose methods were tailored to the chief symptoms of dementia. It also required a new willingness to move beyond existing intellectual boundaries in the quest to understand better the personal and interpersonal contexts in which dementia arises, and to meet the human needs that it generates.

As the world of dementia care opened up to new influences we saw, among others, Tom Kitwood (1990) bringing the insights of social psychology to bear on the interpersonal processes that characterise care; the importation of the theory and practice of sensory integration from the field of learning disabilities; and Bère Miesen (1999) introducing us to the implications for dementia care of advances in the understanding of attachment and loss. It also involved a series of attempts to develop approaches that sought to establish the potential for building therapeutic relationships, utilising interpersonal techniques and skills that address those features of dementia that hinder the maintenance of relationships.

The new enthusiasm for exploring the application of therapeutic approaches from other fields combined with an interest in interpersonal relationships pointed towards the work of the founder of the person-centred therapeutic tradition, Carl Rogers. Person-centred therapy (whose name has, sometimes misleadingly, been appropriated by a host of recent developments in dementia care) is an approach to therapy in which the relationship between therapist and client is seen as the key to therapeutic development. Rogers (1957) described the therapeutic relationship as having six 'necessary and sufficient' features:

'For constructive personality change to occur, it is necessary that these conditions exist and continue over a period of time:
1 Two persons are in psychological contact.
2 The first, whom we shall term the client, is in a stage of incongruence, being vulnerable or anxious.
3 The second person, whom we shall call the therapist, is congruent or integrated in the relationship.
4 The therapist experiences unconditional positive regard for the client.
5 The therapist experiences an empathic understanding of the client's internal frame of reference and endeavors to communicate this experience to the client.
6 The communication to the client of the therapist's empathic understanding and unconditional positive regard is to a minimal degree achieved.'

These features are often summarised – in relation to the role of the therapist – as offering the 'core conditions' of congruence, empathy and (unconditional positive) regard. They have been central to some of the recent attempts to advance the therapeutic standing of interpersonal aspects of dementia care.

Validation therapy

The early writings of the founder of validation therapy, Naomi Feil, contain the first signs of Rogerian ideas gaining a foothold in dementia care. Feil started her career as a group therapist attempting to use the methods of reality orientation, but she became disillusioned at RO's failure to enable her to make contact with group members who had passed beyond the earliest stages of disorientation. Having concluded that this inability was rooted in RO's insistence on presenting the therapist's version of reality, she began to develop an approach (which she later named 'validation') that was based on listening to, and attempting to understand, the seemingly confused speech of people with dementia.

Feil places a strong emphasis on the need for empathy, regard and a genuine approach to those she described as the 'disoriented old-old'. Introducing her reasons for writing *The Validation Breakthrough*, Feil listed her hopes that readers will: '… learn empathy. They will learn to listen and talk with the disoriented instead of restraining them or patronizing them or telling them what to do. They will learn to respect them.' (1993)

Feil developed a number of interpersonal techniques to enhance communication with those at each phase of her own four-stage model of disorientation. Reflective techniques such as repeating key words, rephrasing and mirroring reveal the influence of person-centred therapy and counselling on the practice of validation. After an initial flurry of interest, however, validation has not sustained the impact in Britain that it has had in the USA, Australasia and some parts of the European continent. This has been due in part to British unease with Feil's theory of disorientation, and also her tendency to incorporate elements from other approaches, most notably the psychodynamic traditions. In this country her work served more as encouragement to those who shared her disillusionment with reality orientation, and who were to develop a different way forward.

Resolution therapy

Among the earliest steps were those taken in the first edition of this volume by its editors, Graham Stokes and Fiona Goudie, who challenged validation's psychodynamic explanation of disorientation as an attempt to resolve earlier life crises. Their account of resolution therapy in the chapter 'Counselling Confused Elderly People' suggested that disoriented speech and behaviour were more likely to represent feelings and concerns about the 'here and now'. They recommended that caregivers respond: 'By using the counselling skills of reflective listening, exploration, warmth and acceptance in the tradition of Rogerian humanistic psychology' (1990). Urging an acknowledgement of the feelings being experienced by the confused person and reflecting them in a tentative manner found a resonance with many caregivers who shared validation's willingness to listen, but were uncomfortable with its tendency to make bold interpretations of disoriented speech and behaviour. Although few working in dementia care would describe themselves as 'resolution therapists', many more use those basic counselling skills (gained in the training of many disciplines) in their interactions today as a matter of course.

Pre-therapy

The 'model of meaning and feeling in dementia' put forward by Stokes and Goudie saw the symptoms of dementia as a barrier to contact and communication that resolution sought to overcome. They accepted, however, that eventually that barrier would become insurmountable and '... as dementia progresses, opportunities for counselling or work on acknowledging feelings diminish' (1990). When this stage is reached we can say that the first of Rogers' necessary and sufficient conditions listed above, that: 'Two persons are in psychological contact' is no longer met.

The desire to develop a truly person-centred approach to working with people who have levels of cognitive impairment that inhibit their ability to make psychological contact has led to recent interest being shown in the possible application of pre-therapy with this group (Van Werde & Morton, 1999). pre-therapy was pioneered by Garry Prouty, an American person-centred therapist who was interested in working with client groups previously considered beyond the reach of Rogerian therapy. Prouty was primarily responsible for the evolution of a way of working with those for whom 'psychological contact' is problematic – an approach based on his experience of working with individuals suffering from severe and/or enduring psychosis and with people who have relatively profound learning disabilities. Pre-therapy was initially intended to assist clients and therapists to meet the condition of psychological contact, in order that they may then move on to using person-centred therapy. With the realisation that this would not always be attainable, however, attention became focused on the desirability of achieving and maintaining contact as a goal in itself.

The theoretical basis of Pre-Therapy is simple, perhaps deceptively so. Prouty describes three 'contact functions', which become impaired to varying degrees, in psychosis and in cases involving structural damage to the brain:

- Reality contact – our contact with the world. Awareness of objects, events, place people, etc. When damaged deficits occur with regard to our ability to engage in shared perceptions of reality.
- Affective contact – our contact with ourselves. Awareness of our experience – thoughts, emotions and bodily sensations. When damaged we suffer from an inability to identify our sensations, thoughts and so on as our own and can cease to locate ourselves as the locus of our own experience.
- Communicative contact – our contact with others. Communication of our awareness to others, usually involving the use of language. If damaged we become unable to communicate our experience to others.

The pre-therapy method advocates the use of 'contact reflections' involving the utilisation of reflective techniques similar to those employed in person-centred counselling:

- Situational reflections – to strengthen reality contact. Usually reflections about the client's immediate physical environment and perceptual field: for example, 'The dog is barking', 'The wall is orange', 'Door'.
- Facial reflections – to strengthen affective contact. Usually reflecting the feelings that seem to be communicated by the client's facial expression: 'You look sad', 'You are grinning', 'Your eyes look frightened'.
- Word-for-word reflections – to strengthen communicative contact. Usually reflecting meaningful communication or coherent attempts at communication.

- Body reflections – which consist of physical mirroring of the client's posture or movements, or verbal descriptions of what the client is doing.
- Reiterative reflections – which consist of the repetition of previous reflections that have elicited 'contact behaviours' – ie, those behaviours that are indicative of increased contact functioning.

Prouty describes the desired effect of reflection as: 'Stated simply, reflection intensifies inner feeling to the point that an experiencing process is initiated.' (1976, p1).

The decision as to which kind of reflection is most appropriate in any circumstance will involve considerations about which contact functioning is most in need of strengthening.

Any brief description of the theory and practice of pre-therapy risks creating the impression that it consists of a relatively simple, mechanical use of a set of techniques. In the reality of interacting with the person that shares, at best, only a little of our own perception of reality, the considerations are, of course, far more complex and the art of pre-therapy far more subtle than can be conveyed here (see, for example, Van Werde 1994, pp126–8). Pre-Therapy is realistic about the limits that damage to the client's contact functioning places on our ability to make an empathic response and, in acknowledging this, is the most coherent approach to a genuinely person-centred approach to individuals who are not 'in contact'.

In working with people with dementia who are still able to sustain some degree of psychological contact, there is growing confidence that the kind of reflective responses initiated by validation and resolution therapy can play a valuable role in their care. Person-centred elements, such as those contained in the approaches outlined here, help to redress the 'balance of power' in relationships between the person with dementia and their caregivers. Accounts such as those provided by Tom Kitwood (eg, Kitwood, 1990) of the catastrophic consequences of the imbalances of power that accompany the dementing process persuaded many of the urgent need to do so.

References

Feil N, 1993, *The Validation Breakthrough,* Health Professions Press, Cleveland.

Kitwood T, 1990, 'The Dialectics of Dementia: With Particular Reference to Alzheimer's Disease', *Ageing and Society* 10, pp177–96.

Miesen BML, 1999, *Dementia in close-up,* Routledge, London.

Rogers CR, 1957, 'The Necessary and Sufficient Conditions of Therapeutic Personality Change', *Journal of Consulting Psychology* 21(2), pp95–103.

Stokes G & Goudie F, 1990, 'Counselling Confused Elderly People', in Stokes G & Goudie F(eds), *Working with Dementia,* pp181–90, Speechmark Publishing/Winslow Press, Bicester.

Perrin T, 1997, 'The Positive Response Schedule for Severe Dementia', *Ageing & Mental Health* 1(2), pp184–91.

Prouty G, 1976, 'Pre-Therapy – a Method of Treating Pre-Expressive Psychotic and Retarded Patients', *Psychotherapy: Theory Research and Practice* 13(3), pp290–95.

Van Werde D, 1994, 'Dealing with the Possibility of Psychotic Content in a Seemingly Congruent Communication', Mearns D (ed), *Developing Person Centred Counselling,* pp125–8, Sage, London, 1994.

Van Werde D & Morton I, 1999, 'The relevance of Prouty's Pre-Therapy to dementia care', in Morton I, *Person-Centred Approaches to Dementia Care,* pp139–66, Speechmark Publishing/Winslow Press, Bicester.

Further reading

Feil N, 1992, *V/F Validation: The Feil Method* (revised 2nd edn), Feil Productions, Cleveland.

Kitwood T, 1997, *Dementia Reconsidered,* Open University Press, Buckingham.

Morton I, 1999, *Person-Centred Approaches to Dementia Care,* Speechmark Publishing/Winslow Press, Bicester.

Prouty G, 1994, *Theoretical Evolutions in Person-Centered/Experiential Therapy,* Praeger, Westport.

CHAPTER 17

Working with Psychological Distress

Fiona Goudie

PSYCHOLOGICAL DISTRESS IS COMMON throughout the course of dementia. Depression and anxiety are the most likely psychological responses. One in five people with early dementia will experience depression, and symptoms of anxiety are more common than this. Other difficulties can include:

- Avoidance of social situations and fears about leaving home or being separated from a partner.
- 'Obsessive' behaviour (associated with repeated checking and trying to do things correctly).
- Psychotic symptoms (involving delusions and hallucinations).
- Symptoms of post-traumatic stress (which may lead to remembering and reliving traumatic events from earlier in life, such as abuse or war trauma).

These can all occur independently and may be mistaken for dementia. In this chapter, the main causes and consequences of psychological distress for the person with dementia are discussed. Psychological interventions are described and recommendations are made for implementation in practice. Trauma and dementia are not covered in this chapter, but are the focus of Chapter 18.

Causes and consequences of psychological ill-being

Some of the main causes of psychological ill-being in dementia are summarised in Table 17.1. It would be surprising if a person coping with dementia did not experience emotional reactions to these experiences. Sadness at a diagnosis of dementia; anxiety about how to cope with memory and other difficulties; fear of being embarrassed socially for forgetting names, and the adoption of rituals to make the structure of the day feel safer are normal reactions to coping with the losses and changes of dementia.

However, a combination of biological, psychological and social factors can exacerbate these reactions and lead to additional distress.

Interventions

There is now a wide range of psychological interventions that are effective for older people. Some of these have been modified for people with dementia, and others specifically developed for them.

Validation and resolution therapy

Validation therapy (Feil, 1992; see also Morton, Chapter 16 this volume) was developed as a client-centred approach for listening to and understanding the apparently confused speech of people with dementia. Interpretation is linked to Feil's model of disorientation and the possibility of unresolved earlier life crises.

Resolution therapy (Goudie & Stokes, 1989; Stokes & Goudie, 1990) also emphasises the use of counselling skills (reflective listening, exploration, warmth and acceptance) to try to understand and respond to what the person with dementia might be feeling. The focus is on what is going on in the here and now. So, for example, if someone was insisting they must go home to cook their husband's tea (even though he has been dead for many years), the worker would *accept* that the person had been thinking about their husband, and would *reflect* this ('So you've been thinking about your husband and the meals you used to cook this afternoon?') while trying to *explore* what the current feelings behind this are ('It's very quiet here today, are you feeling bored?'), and *resolve* them ('Would you like to give me a hand with the tea trolley?').

Table 17.1 *Causes and consequences of psychological ill-being in dementia*

Causes of distress	Consequences
Biological	
Changes in cells and biochemistry of the central nervous system.	Anxiety, panic, depression, hallucinations and delusions.
Changes to cortical and subcortical brain structures that control emotions.	As above. Can also lead to apparently 'flat' mood and lack of motivation.
Effects of drug and alcohol toxicity.	Excessive arousal or depression, acute confusion, hallucinations, paranoia.
Psychological	
Impact of diagnosis and experience of living with chronic illness.	Anger, disbelief, sadness, fear.
Impact of changing relationships with family.	Loneliness, sadness, depression, frustration.
Changes in effectiveness of coping strategies.	Anxiety, panic, obsessional behaviour.
Increased negative cognitions about self, world and future.	Depression, feeling worthless.
Reduction in pleasurable reinforcing activities and thoughts.	Isolation, sadness, depression.
Learned helplessness associated with disempowering attitudes of others to people with dementia.	Depression, despair.
Impact of sudden crises (bereavement, illness, move to residential care).	Panic, reactivation of feelings associated with earlier traumas, searching for parents, hallucinations.
Lack of a sense of attachment to a significant person.	Fear, loneliness.
Social	
Impact of negative social attitudes.	Physical and emotional isolation.
Disempowering nature of assessment and service delivery.	Anger, sadness, feeling out of control. Avoidance of services.
Reduced social contact and relationships for people with dementia and their families.	Anxiety and depression for carers and people with dementia, early breakdown in relationship and ability to care.
Poverty, gender and class factors leading to inequalities in access to financial support, good care and treatment.	Untreated distress and unsupported carers where access to good care is poor.

These approaches emphasise the importance of the emotional life of people with dementia. By using them routinely, those working in dementia care can help yo promote psychological wellbeing as well as establishing a basis for positive relationships on which to offer more focused help if it is needed.

Reminiscence and life review

Until the 1960s, reminiscence was seen as a negative activity, likely to overemphasise past events and potentially cause distress to older people. Butler (1963) saw life review and related reminiscence activities as normative and undertaken by most people.

Reminiscence methods are used for a wide range of purposes including oral history, enhancing social contact, maintaining old skills, improving cross-generational and cultural understanding, life review, therapy, and for fun (see Bender *et al*, 1999 for a summary of purposes). Reminiscence activities are usually carried out in groups, but can happen on an individual basis. They are increasingly used with people who have dementia. The rationale for this has been that remote memories of childhood and early adulthood are relatively well preserved until later in the course of dementia. Drawing on these memories can help the person maintain a sense of themselves as a person and enable them to feel confidence in some areas of memory, even if day-to-day events are difficult to recall. Open-ended discussion around particular themes (such as childhood, first job or family life) may be a useful approach with people who have few cognitive impairments. However, it is more common to use a range of triggers to stimulate recall. These commonly include music, video tapes, photographic material and everyday objects of historical interest. Drama, art and literary projects may also have reminiscence as the focus. Some approaches involve individuals writing, using tapes or diaries.

Bender *et al* (1999) emphasise the importance of staff 'doing their homework' in advance by getting an individual life history of the clients they will involve in reminiscence. Goudie and Stokes (1990), in the same vein, discuss the importance of individual reminiscence profiles. This information is needed to ensure that the subject matter is something with which people will be familiar. Those who conduct reminiscence need to be confident about using a variety of stimulus material, and have good non-verbal as well as verbal communication skills. In addition, those running groups need good groupwork skills, and to be able to involve people with a range of cognitive abilities. At least two facilitators will be needed for a group of six. Certain people may not benefit from a group approach. Compulsive reminiscers (who may have unresolved feelings about an earlier life event) can dominate a group unhelpfully, and some people have no real interest in reminiscing. For others certain topics, if introduced without thought or awareness of the individual's life history, can trigger distress (for example, playing the sound of an air-raid siren for someone who experienced bombing during a war). Overall, however, such groups appear to be stimulating and enjoyable to those who participate, and increase staff awareness of the lives of the people they care for. Research into group reminiscence for specific problems like depression is in its infancy, and a more structured approach that incorporates specific psychotherapeutic principles, may be required (Fry, 1983).

Life-story work involves looking back over the past – usually on a one-to-one basis. It does not set out to resolve past or present problems, but can be used to help families and carers gain greater understanding of the person they care for; to have something for families to pass on to carers if someone moves into a residential setting, and to orientate the person to the reality of their life. Some work can take the form of a life-story book, with sections arranged decade by decade through the person's life, but could also be a visual record of photos and memorabilia. Murphy (1994) describes good practice with people who have dementia.

Life review is a more focused and structured approach. The therapist and older person are usually working one-to-one on 'conflict resolution … self-acceptance and coming to terms with life' (Garland, 1994). The technique of recalling specific events and re-evaluating them may involve painful experiences. It is a psychotherapeutic approach requiring a trained therapist with access to supervision. Generally, life review has been used with people who are not dementing, whereas reminiscence has a wider application.

As with validation and resolution therapies, services which encourage staff and clients to share experiences, maintain skills and enjoy the company of others can promote wellbeing without trying to undertake group psychotherapy in the absence of training or supervision.

Coping with the diagnosis

The feelings associated with receiving a diagnosis of dementia are similar to those associated with a diagnosis of cancer or other terminal illness, and with bereavement and loss. For professional staff, giving a diagnosis and discussing implications can be stressful and may generate feelings of panic, a desire to avoid the subject or pass on the task to someone they believe to be better qualified at dealing with bad news.

In services that deal specifically with early diagnosis and its treatment, such as a memory clinic, the team may have developed their skills in pre- and post-diagnostic counselling (see Chapter 5). Grief counselling and therapy models such as that set out by Worden (1992) can be valuable in relation to the post-diagnostic counselling work. However, many people with dementia never receive a diagnosis in the early stages of their disease. As their condition progresses they attend hospitals or day centres with other people who are obviously forgetful and have communication difficulties. Yet it is unusual for the treatment programmes in these settings to address directly the diagnosis and associated feelings for their service-users. One example of a user-initiated approach to this is summarised in Case Study 17.1.

Case Study 17.1 Why we're here – coping with forgetting

The Lawns was a newly opened day hospital for people with dementia. The therapeutic programme included reminiscence groups, general knowledge and word quizzes, social activities and skill-building (such as gardening or cooking). Staff were keen to find out what attenders thought of this programme and conducted interviews with a number of them. Some of the comments made included: 'I don't know why I'm here – I think my husband wants rid of me.' 'I've been told I've got Alzheimer's and it would help coming here, but no one's told me what will help.' 'Everyone is confused here, will I get like that?'

A number of attenders were interested in attending a group on 'Why we're here – coping with forgetting.' The group had six participants and was run by an OT and a psychologist for 10 weeks. Early sessions were information-orientated, but became more unstructured as participants

---

gained confidence in talking about their feelings of sadness about being denied information on their illness; anger at collusion between carers and professionals, and their fears and hopes for the future. The group leaders were struck by the levels of support and problem-solving offered by group members to each other about marital tensions, loss of friendships and nursing home admission.

The group was difficult to evaluate in a quantitative way, but a number of qualitative changes were observed. Members preferred attending the group to other diversional activities. One commented, 'I've found people I can be honest with.' A husband said 'When she comes home after the group she is much more talkative.' The social worker of one client remarked that she had been in a 'stalemate' situation with the man and his family over residential care admission. 'But after attending the group he told his wife he thought he'd be less of a burden to her if he went for respite.'

There were some needs for staff arising from the group. In their peer supervision they spent more time discussing group process issues and the feelings evoked in themselves than they did in response to the other groups they ran.

Anxiety and phobic reactions

Anxiolytics have frequently been the first choice by the general practitioner or mental health team in treating an anxious older person – whether or not they have dementia. Yet psychological interventions such as relaxation training are effective with older people (Scogin *et al*, 1992), and avoid some of the unwanted side-effects associated with anxiolytics, such as over sedation and risk of falling. The ABC approach described by Stokes (Chapter 8) can be used to understand the factors contributing to and maintaining anxiety. Questionnaires like the Hospital Anxiety and Depression Scale can be used to help distinguish anxiety from depression.

People in the early stages of dementia can be helped to use cognitive, behavioural and anxiety-management strategies if these are modified to take account of memory and information-processing difficulties. For example, tapes of brief relaxation techniques and breathing exercises can be used on a personal stereo after regular practice with someone skilled at demonstrating them. Carers can be trained to use the technique alongside the person with dementia. Physical exercise and the use of distraction techniques (such as listening to music or focusing attention on objects in the room) may be valuable, but will need to be reinforced by writing them down or by using a family member or carer to remind the person to use them.

Apparent phobic reactions include the avoidance of social situations and a reluctance to leave home or loved ones. Such a reaction can be part of an understandable response to a change in one's ability to participate in or enjoy an activity. For some people, what is most important is being able to withdraw from a social occasion or give up an activity with dignity rather than fearing ridicule.

However, for the person who wants to overcome their anxieties, principles of graded exposure and encouraging mastery over small tasks before moving on to bigger ones can be used (see Case Study 17.2). This is likely to be important when someone has become socially isolated over a period of time and services are trying to engage them in new activities or day centres.

Case Study 17.2 Mrs Choudry copes with panic

Mrs Choudhry had been living with her daughter, son-in-law and grandchildren for 10 years. Initially she had enjoyed looking after her grandchildren and helping with the shopping and household chores. Her memory and ability to cope with chores and childcare had worsened over the last two to three years. She had stopped going to the market and retreated to her bedroom if visitors called to see her. On a couple of occasions she had a panic attack when visitors called unexpectedly. Her GP involved the Community Mental Health Team for Older People. A full assessment confirmed a diagnosis of probable Alzheimer's disease. Of particular concern to her community psychiatric nurse (CPN) was the panic and anxiety she experienced during the assessment process. The CPN was able to show Mrs Choudhry and her daughter controlled breathing and relaxation techniques to cope with panic. She then helped them compile a list of people and places that Mrs Choudhry had been

---

avoiding. She did want to keep contact with members of her extended family, so they came up with a list of social contacts going from those she felt most able to cope with to those she felt least able to cope with. Mrs Choudhry and her daughter worked gradually, using relaxation to help her cope with a planned 10-minute visit from a close relative, eventually working up to a meal with a cousin's family.

Mrs Choudhry's dementia did not improve, but with regular reminders to 'do her breathing' before visits from certain close family members, she was able to remain in the sitting room and enjoy their company.

Because the person with dementia has impaired memory for learning new skills, it is likely that helpful strategies will need to be reinforced continually by a carer, rather than expecting the person to remember what to do themselves.

Depression

Depression is frequently unrecognised and untreated among older people. However, it can be a significant problem among people with dementia, their carers and those who live in residential settings. Antidepressants can be helpful in treating the biological symptoms of depression (such as sleep, appetite disurbance or psychomotor retardation), and these are discussed in Chapter 19. Psychological approaches to treating depression are increasingly applied in work with older clients. Cognitive behaviour therapy has one of the strongest evidence bases and has been used with people with dementia (Teri & Gallagher-Thompson, 1991). Behavioural techniques may focus on identifying events that the person has pleasure in and control over (see Case Study 17.3). These are often reduced in people with dementia. Developing strategies to increase control over and pleasure in events can be helpful.

Case Study 17.3 Mr Walker's control and pleasure chart

Mr Walker was 78 years old and lived on his own, having been widowed 10 years ago. He had a two-year history of memory impairment and a three-month history of depression. The depression seemed to have worsened since he started to have home care to enable him to attend a day hospital twice weekly. The home carer helped him to dress in time for the transport to the day hospital and collected his pension, did some shopping and meal preparation. As part of his assessment at the day hospital the OT helped him complete a control and pleasure chart. (There is an extract from this in Figure 17.1.)

Day/time	Event	Control rating (1=low;10=high)	Pleasure rating (1=low;10=high)
Tues 8.00	Home carer helping me wash and dress. (Feel rushed)	3	1
9.00–9.30	Eat breakfast got ready by carer. Not what I usually have.	1	2
9.30–10.00	Wait for transport. (Would usually go to get a paper at corner shop)	1	1

Figure 17.1 *Control- and pleasure-rating*

The therapist also asked him what he was feeling about these events. Together they noted down common thoughts and feelings in a notebook during the next few sessions. (Figure 17.2 shows extracts from the notebook.)

Day/time	Situation	Feelings	Thoughts
Tues 8.00	Home carer helping me wash and dress	Ashamed	I must be useless now
9.00	Eat tea and toast. Usually have coffee and cereal	Angry	I can never have what I want any more
10.00	Waiting for transport	Frightened	Maybe they're going to put me in a home

Figure 17.2 *Thoughts and feelings record sheet*

For Mr Walker, the experience of dementia was being made worse by the form of support he was receiving. His sense of control over his life was being eroded. He was experiencing negative thoughts about himself ('I must be useless now'), his world and his future ('I can never have what I want anymore'). Although it would be unrealistic for Mr Walker to think he would never need more support, his current circumstances and thoughts were unnecessarily negative. They were making him feel angry, fearful and ashamed. He was beginning to withdraw from the positive relationships in his life (children and friends who understood his difficulties, but wanted to enjoy time with him).

His therapist was able to work with him and the home carer to ensure that he had more control over his morning routine. She helped him find alternative ways of thinking about his situation. He sometimes forgot what they discussed in therapy, but after about six weeks he began to make the following remarks. 'I know it's not me that's useless – my illness makes me forget things, I've got to make allowances.' and 'Anna (daughter) is taking me shopping now, so I've got plenty of the food I want.' His mood had improved on the scale used by the day-hospital team.

It was important not to trivialise or minimise the significance of dementia for Mr Walker, but it was possible to reduce unneccessary depression and distress using cognitive-behavioural therapy.

Psychodynamic approaches

There has been a growing interest in the application of psychodynamic approaches to work with older people (Knight, 1996). Terry (1997) has written movingly about their use with people who have dementia and their carers. He sees the aim of this work as helping the client resolve unconscious internal conflict underlying suffering and distress. While this approach may be thought of as particularly useful for people who have recently been given a diagnosis, Terry describes its application (through paying attention to his own responses and feelings) with a man who had severe dysphasia and 'behaviour problems'. He also describes support groups for staff to think about their own and their patients' feelings about being in an institutional setting, and to help them understand that some of their own feelings may be unconscious communications from their patients.

Conclusions and recommendations

Many of the psychological interventions discussed in this chapter have been developed for other populations, and have been modified for people with dementia by taking account of the attention, memory, language and problem-solving difficulties they may have. This means that so far there is limited research evidence for their effectiveness. However, the case studies have attempted to illustrate some of the emerging findings from clinical practice. It is hoped that further application of these approaches will help develop the evidence base.

References

Bender M, Bauckham P & Norris A, 1999, 'The Therapeutic Purposes of Reminiscence', Sage, London.

Butler RN, 1963, 'The Life Review: An Interpretation of Reminiscence in the Aged', *Psychiatry* 26, pp65–76.

Feil N, 1992 *Validation: The Feil method* (revised 2nd edn), Feil Productions, Cleveland.

Fry PS, 1983, 'Structured and unstructured reminiscence training and depression among the elderly,' *Clinical Gerontologist* 1, pp15–37.

Garland J, 1994, 'What splendour it all coheres: Life review therapy with older people', in Bornat J (ed), *Reminiscence Reviewed: Perspectives, evaluations, achievements*, Open University Press, Buckingham.

Goudie F & Stokes G, 1990, 'Reminiscence with dementia sufferers', in Stokes G & Goudie F, *Working with Dementia*, pp121–7, Speechmark Publishing/Winslow Press, Bicester.

Kitwood T & Bredin K, 1992, *Person to Person*, Gale Centre Publications, Loughton.

Kitwood T, 1997, *Dementia Reconsidered*, Open University Press, Buckingham.

Murphy C J, 1994, *'It started with a sea-shell': Life Story Work and People with Dementia*, University of Stirling, Stirling.

Scogin F, Rickard HC, Keith S, Wilson J & McElreath, L, 1992, 'Progressive and imaginal relaxation training for elderly persons with subjective anxiety', *Psychology and Ageing* 7, pp419–24.

Stokes G & Goudie F, 1990 'Counselling confused elderly people', Stokes G & Goudie F, *Working with Dementia*, pp181–90, Speechmark Publishing/Winslow Press, Bicester.

Teri L & Gallagher-Thompson D, 1991, 'Cognitive-behavioural interventions for treatment of depression in Alzheimer's patients', *Gerontologist,* 31, pp413–16.

Terry P, 1997, *Counselling the Elderly and their Carers*, Macmillan Press, London.

Knight B, 1996, *Psychotherapy with Older Adults* (2nd edn), Sage, Beverly Hills, California.

Worden W, 1992, *Grief Counselling and Grief Therapy* (2nd edn), Springer, New York.

CHAPTER 18

Trauma and Dementia

Fiona Goudie

TRAUMA CAN OCCUR THROUGHOUT life and can take many forms. It can be caused directly by others (as in violence and emotional abuse); by neglect (such as lack of parental nurturing), or through circumstances beyond anyone's direct control (eg, war, earthquakes, or untreatable illness).

The individual usually has no power, support or protection against the traumatic event. The circumstances can lead to fear, apathy and aggression. This description of the individual's situation and their response is common in dementia. Dementia can be viewed as a traumatic event in itself *and* as a condition that changes someone's capacity to cope with other traumatic situations they have experienced.

This chapter considers examples of both these types of trauma and discusses ways of helping people deal with their experiences. It begins by considering early attachment and the effect this can have on later reactions to stressful circumstances.

The importance of early attachment

Why do people differ in their apparent capacity to cope with stressful events? One explanation is that people differ in the way they are able to form and make use of secure, stable 'attachment relationships'. The concept of attachment was originally described by psychoanalysts such as Bowlby (1969). Attachment to a caregiver has survival value and ensures the child's safety and security. Attachment *behaviour* occurs when safety and security are threatened, and includes searching, clinging to and calling out for the caregiver. The way in which parents meet their child's attachment needs will determine their attachment style for life. Threatened or actual abandonment, separations and abuse in childhood can affect the individual's personality, their capacity for forming relationships, and emotional reactions at times of stress in adulthood.

In the last decade there has been an increase in research on adult patterns of attachment (see Rutter [1995] for a review). Symptoms of anxiety associated with separation – Separation Anxiety Disorder (SAD), which is a recognised childhood disorder – are more easily masked in adulthood, but may present as agoraphobia or panic disorder and be inappropriately treated. It is suggested that the capacity to cope with grief can be significantly affected by childhood attachment style.

For someone with dementia, experiencing loss (perhaps of former roles, abilities, relationships, of their home and ultimately the self that once was) can severely challenge their feelings of safety and security. Magai and Passman (1997), in a study of emotional expression in dementia, found that people with secure attachment patterns before developing dementia had more positive emotional expression, and that expressed hostility among dementia sufferers was associated with premorbidly hostile behaviour. They argue that attachment style and personality should be considered more fully when trying to understand problem behaviours in dementia. They have particular relevance when events from the person's earlier life were very traumatic. The significance of this is highlighted in Case Study 18.1.

Case Study 18.1 Mrs Taylor's anxious attachment style

Mrs Taylor, aged 76, had a five-year history of probable Alzheimer's disease. She lived with her husband who was 82 and physically frail, with severe arthritis, but devoted to caring for his wife. The couple's only son lived some distance away, and came to stay for a couple of days every three or four weeks. Mrs Taylor's memory was very poor for recent events. She was unable to cook or carry out domestic chores alone and needed a lot of prompting from her husband to dress and wash herself. She attended a day centre twice a week. Sometimes she was interested in the morning activities – especially if she could get involved in baking. By lunchtime she was usually walking round the centre asking for her husband, and by mid afternoon she was physically grabbing members of staff and pleading with them to find him. She was often very angry with her husband when she got home and had hit him on one or two occasions.

As Mr Taylor's arthritis worsened, he was unable to help his wife dress or wash. A home help was arranged. However, when the carer tried to help her with washing and dressing she lashed out, kicking and hitting and refusing assistance.

The social worker involved with Mrs Taylor wondered whether medication would be needed to control her behaviour, and arranged a meeting with Mr Taylor and their son to discuss this and residential care options. During the meeting a lot of information about Mrs Taylor was disclosed. She had been physically abused as a child by both parents. She married Mr Taylor – her first boyfriend – at the age of 17. Throughout their marriage she had been jealous of any female colleagues he had at work and was nervous of women callers to the house.

It appeared that a life-long anxious attachment style and the type of support being offered increased her fears that her husband was abandoning her. Mrs Taylor was offered some home-based respite rather than day care twice a week. This involved an outreach worker taking her and two other clients for walks or shopping and rotating a cookery session in their homes. She seemed to feel less threatened by this than attending the day centre. It was important to offer some blocks of overnight respite on a regular basis to give Mr Taylor a break from helping his wife with personal care tasks. He was keen to visit his wife daily, thereby minimising her fears that he had left her. He and their son also made some tapes, reminiscing about their lives together, which were used nightly to help Mrs Taylor settle (Simulated Presence Therapy, see p200) during the respite periods.

Attachment and parent fixation

Miesen has defined 'parent fixation' (1992) to describe someone with dementia who believes one or both parents is alive when they have been dead for some years. Attachment behaviours characteristic of parent fixation include trying to go home; asking where/how parents are; wanting to behave in line with parental expectations, and believing they are back in the family home.

While psychiatrists have defined 'parent fixation' as confabulations or delusions linked to organic change and cognitive deterioration, Miesen argues that the emotional experience of dementia is a 'strange situation', exacerbated by hospital or residential care settings. Dementia activates attachment behaviours, and parent fixation can be viewed as an expression of the need for safety and security. Although Miesen's model is based on small-scale research, it is a valuable contribution to the psychosocial understanding of dementia – particularly in relation to behaviours that have traditionally been viewed as organic in origin, with drug treatment as the preferred method of management.

Reactivation of traumatic experiences

Post-traumatic stress disorder has become increasingly recognised as a psychological consequence of war for service veterans and for many civilians living through war. Specific symptoms include flashbacks, intrusive thoughts, auditory and visual re-experiencing of traumatic events, nightmares and the tendency to be easily aroused or startled.

For many older people who have experienced trauma in earlier life, avoidance of memories has been made possible for many years by engaging in physically demanding activities, working long hours, and using tobacco and alcohol. However, late life losses associated with bereavement, reduction in physical ability and early dementia can lead to the reactivation of traumatic memories that have been successfully repressed for many years.

Case Study 18.2 illustrates an example of this and describes an intervention.

Case Study 18.2 Mr Czarnocka relieves his wartime experiences

Mr Czarnocka was an 84-year-old Pole who had been resident in The Elms for six months since the death of his wife. A combination of severe arthritis and moderate memory problems had made it difficult for him to look after himself in his own home. Staff at The Elms were concerned about his behaviour. He was hostile to staff and would remove food from other residents' plates at meal times and hoard it in drawers and cupboards in his room. He was reluctant to eat his own meal in public. He appeared frightened of going to sleep, and when he did go to bed he wanted to use the furniture to barricade himself into his room.

The head of the home and a visiting CPN were able to develop enough of a relationship with Mr Czarnocka and one of his daughters to find out that he had been a prisoner of war. He described how he survived starvation and death in the camp. He stayed awake at night to ensure his possessions were not stolen, and sought out and then hid any rations uneaten by the ill or dying. He had not talked about these experiences for decades, but the communal eating situation in the home and the noise of other residents and staff at night reactivated some of the old fears and behaviours. Before the onset of Alzheimer's disease, he had been able to distract himself from certain memories by reading and watching TV late at night. His concentration now affected his enjoyment of these activities.

A number of strategies helped Mr Czarnocka and those caring for him to cope better with his traumatic memories and reactions. The CPN suggested making a life-story notice-board with some of his mementoes and photographs. The board included recent photos of his children and grandchildren, and information about work and hobbies as well as war and pre-war mementoes. It had two functions. It reminded staff of Mr Czarnocka's Polish background and prisoner-of-war experiences and enabled them to empathise with him more readily. It also helped them to ground him in the here and now by drawing his attention to photos of his grandchildren, his long-service award from the local steelworks and his membership card for the Polish Club he still attended occasionally with his son. His hoarding of food was reduced by giving him meals on his own in his bedroom. He began to stay up late in the lounge with one or two other residents who enjoyed late-night TV. As far as possible, the same two keyworkers on nights would help him get into bed. They would regularly repeat a conversation about the here and now, which included a reminder of the date, current news, any recent or planned visitors, who they were, and that they would be looking after him and his belongings overnight.

Some difficulties remained, particularly when staff changed, but Mr Czarnocka felt much more settled and the home felt more able to cope on a day-to-day basis.

Dementia and dementia care can cause trauma

The progressive cognitive impairments associated with dementia and the impact this has on the individual's abilities, social relationships and self-esteem can be very traumatic. When these are combined with service models that ignore the emotional experience of the individual; collude to avoid discussing what is going on, and provide task-centred care the effects can be devastating.

Some people with dementia are traumatised in the *here and now* by the nature of their experiences or the inadequacy of the care they are receiving. Sadly it is often the most vulnerable, being looked after in institutional settings with poor care regimes, who may be at greatest risk of physical, emotional and sexual abuse. Traumatic reactions are not always a response to earlier life experience, and requests to go home may reflect upset with current care and relationships rather than 'parent fixation'. Services that seek out and value user views, employ methods like Dementia Care Mapping when people cannot speak for themselves, and encourage staff appraisal and development will have an improved capacity to identify potentially abusive and traumatic practices in current care settings.

Strategies for supporting traumatic experiences

Examples of how staff can support people who are experiencing the effects of trauma are described in the two case studies above. It is important for staff working with people with dementia to have access to relevant information about an individual's history. They need to understand how changes to the way a person is cared for, their environment, their relationships and loss (eg, bereavements or carers leaving) can have a traumatic effect. Some important considerations and strategies for supporting people through traumatic (and potentially traumatic) experiences are summarised below.

- Help maintain meaning of personal possessions. Photos, objects, clothes and furniture form significant links to the person's recent and longer-term past. They can be comforting and reassuring for someone making the transition to long-term care. However, the importance of the possessions may be forgotten over time. Carers need to be active in documenting why an object was brought and what it means, and maintaining discussion about the meaning.
- Simulated presence therapy (Woods & Ashley, 1995). This involves playing a tape of the voices of family members. This could take the form of an audio letter or diary. It may be valuable for those who are agitated or searching out loved ones, as in Case Study 18.1 above.
- Encouraging grief and loss work. Use counselling or therapy if appropriate (Worden, 1991), and consider creative therapies – for example, music therapy (Bright, 1992; Aldridge, 2000) for clients who have difficulty expressing themselves verbally. Bright describes how the planned use of music can help people achieve non-musical goals. Intact cortical functions may be more readily accessed through music, and adverse effects of partial aphasia may be lifted. While music may evoke tears and sadness, it does not in itself make a person unhappy. According to Bright it can 'take the lid off' what was below the surface, and ventilation of these feelings can bring a sense of relief.
- Pay attention to times of transition (such as dealing with diagnosis, beginning to use day or respite services, or moving into residential care). These times are likely to be associated with the strongest feelings of abandonment or re-awakening of earlier responses to trauma. Support with the adjustment to the new experience should be available to everyone at these times. People who have been identified as having a particularly traumatic past may need specific counselling or therapy.
- Life-story work. For example, in Case Study 18.2, Mr Czarnocka was eventually able to share some of his experiences as a prisoner of war

with the staff in The Elms. They had some understanding that he was feeling very anxious and threatened during the times when he tried to remove food from other residents' plates. They could use other approaches like resolution therapy to acknowledge that these feelings were being triggered by the present circumstances and find an alternative solution. Life-story work has its origins in work with children in care. A useful summary of format, content and use is provided by Murphy and Moyes (1997). The important point is that the life-story is not necessarily a 'book' kept in a filing cabinet. It can involve using tapes, photos, display boards or objects in a memory box. The work should be seen as part of an ongoing proces to be used, not locked away when it is finished.

- Coping strategies for managing panic and anxiety. People in the early stages of dementia can be helped to use cognitive, behavioural and anxiety-management strategies if these are modified to take account of memory and information-processing difficulties. For example, tapes of brief relaxation techniques and breathing exercises can be used on a personal stereo after regular practice with someone skilled at demonstrating them. Identifying and using helpful distraction techniques (eg, listening to music, counting cars or ceiling tiles) will need to be reinforced by writing them down, or by using a family member or carer to remind the person to use them.

- Creating a containing therapeutic environment, which supports staff in being 'significant others' to people with dementia. This goes beyond the idea of a key worker and acknowledges that both workers and people with dementia can have powerful feelings (positive and negative) for each other. Good supervision that pays attention to these feelings can help staff manage the intensity of emotion that often surrounds working with people with dementia, as well as avoiding traumatic reactions for clients caused by abrupt discharges or transfers of care.

References

Aldridge D (ed), 2000, *Music Therapy in Dementia Care*, Jessica Kingsley, London.

Bowlby J, 1969, *Attachment and Loss: Vol 1: Attachment*, Basic Books, New York.

Bright R, 1992, 'Music Therapy in the Management of Dementia', in Jones G and Miesen B (eds), *Care-giving in Dementia: Research and Applications*, Routledge, London.

Magai C & Passman V, 1997, 'The interpersonal basis of emotional behaviour and emotional regulation', in Lawton MP and Schaie KW (eds), *Annual Review of Gerontology and Geriatrics* 17, Springer, New York.

Miesen B, 1992, 'Attachment theory and dementia', in Jones A and Miesen B, (1993), *Caregiving in Dementia, Vol 1*, Routledge, London.

Murphy C & Moyes M, 1997, 'Life story work', in Marshall M (ed), *State of the Art in Dementia Care*, Centre for Policy on Ageing, London.

Rutter M, 1995, 'Clinical implications of attachment concepts: retrospect and prospect', *Journal of Child Psychology and Psychiatry* 36(4), pp549–71.

Woods P & Ashley J, 1995, 'Simulated presence therapy: Using selected memories to manage problem behaviours in Alzheimer's Disease patients', *Geriatric Nursing* 16(1), pp9–14.

Worden W, 1991, *Grief Counselling and Grief Therapy,* 2nd edn, Routledge, London.

CHAPTER 19

Medication in the Treatment of Dementia

John Wattis

The medical approach to dementia

Medical practice emphasises treatment based on good evidence and the importance of the doctor-patient relationship in delivering that treatment. The diagnostic approach is concerned with recognising patterns of disease so that appropriate treatment can be agreed. A diagnosis is essentially a hypothesis about what is wrong with the patient. It is based on the concept that, by listening to the history, examining the patient and performing necessary investigations, diseases can be identified and named. These diseases are generally due to genetic or environmental factors or infection, or a mixture of different causes. Understanding the causes of disease enables rational treatment to be planned. In psychiatry, causes are often multiple and the approach to treatment therefore has to take into account many factors. Diagnosis is particularly important where specific treatment is available. Since the first edition of this book, drugs have been licensed for the treatment of Alzheimer's disease, and differential diagnosis of the various causes of dementia (see Chapter 2) is now more important than it was.

The pathology of dementia

After death, examination of a brain damaged by Alzheimer's disease shows some shrinkage and microscopic lesions known as senile plaques and neurofibrillary tangles, often in great abundance. The brain's chemical messengers, known as neurotransmitters, are also depleted, especially acetylcholine. This discovery led to hopes that some kind of replacement therapy analogous to the use of L-dopa to replace dopamine in Parkinson's disease might be of use. Dietary supplementation with choline proved to be of little or no use, but another strategy based on acetylcholine depletion was to block its breakdown in the body by inhibiting the enzymes responsible for this. Thus the first class of anti-Alzheimer's drugs – the acetylcholinesterase inhibitors – was developed (see below).

Vascular (or 'multi-infarct') dementia is related to stroke illness and high blood pressure. Smoking, unhealthy diet, being overweight and all the factors that increase the risk of stroke also increase the risk of multi-infarct dementia. Attention to prevention, not only through 'life-style' measures, but also through the treatment of high blood pressure is very worthwhile. Aspirin in very low doses (75 mg per day) may also help in prevention by reducing the liability of the blood to form clots. Some antidepressants, especially the Serotonin Specific Reuptake Inhibitors (SSRIs) may also reduce the tendency of the blood to form clots as a 'side-effect' to their main action.

Depression should also be mentioned. A degree of depression may affect up to a fifth of people with early dementia. Depression is approximately twice as common in people with early dementia as it is in people without the diagnosis.

Principles of prescribing

Like any other management, prescription should only follow a careful assessment. It is essential to distinguish between the specific use of a drug to treat or interfere with the processes of a disease (eg, antibiotics in pneumonia or acetylcholinesterase inhibitors in Alzheimer's disease) and symptomatic use (eg, to induce sleep or reduce 'aggressive' behaviour). In specific use, medical prescription is more easily justified, though other measures (eg, physiotherapy for pneumonia, carer education and support in dementia) are often important. In symptomatic use, however, the alternatives may often be preferable to medication, especially when the side-effects of medication outweigh the benefits.

Once prescription has been decided on as part of a more general treatment plan, another principle – that of minimal effective medication – is vital. Because medication often has unwanted as well as beneficial effects, it is essential that the minimum number of drugs are prescribed in the lowest effective dose for the shortest time necessary to produce the desired effects. Issuing repeat prescriptions for sleeping tablets can be harmful to old people, who may suffer unwanted effects as a result of medication that is too prolonged. Sometimes brain function may be improved by stopping inappropriate medication as well as by starting new treatment.

Psychotropic medication

Drugs that primarily affect the mind are known as psychotropic (literally mind-changing). Some (eg, opium) have been known and used for thousands of years, but the modern range of psychotropic drugs has only been developed over the last 50 years. Psychotropics were traditionally divided into three main groups, according to their main mode of action: antidepressants, antipsychotics and anxiolytics. To this we can now add the category of anti-dementia drugs.

Anti-dementia drugs

Acetylcholine is the main neurotransmitter that is depleted in Alzheimer's disease. Three drugs, which prevent the breakdown of this chemical in the brain, have so far been licensed in the UK and others will probably follow. Donepezil (Aricept), Galantamine (Reminyl), and Rivastigmine (Exelon) have been shown to produce small but statistically significant improvements in memory. They should only be prescribed by specialists, and at present not all health authorities have agreed to fund their use. Generally, where they are used, guidelines are followed that mean that if the patient does not show definite benefit within three months, the medication is discontinued. Under these conditions, about 30 to 40 per cent of selected patients continue treatment beyond three months and this group often shows benefit in activities of daily living that is apparent to relatives, as well as improvement in performance on memory tests. Those who do respond generally need to continue on treatment for a long time.

Other classes of anti-dementia drugs are being developed. Over the next 10 to 20 years there are hopes that drugs will be found that can interfere with the underlying processes of Alzheimer's disease and vascular dementia. If and when such drugs become available, very early diagnosis will become extremely important so that people can start taking the medication before symptoms of dementia develop. No discussion of anti-dementia drugs would be complete without mention of Gingko Biloba. This herbal remedy has been shown to have some effect in Alzheimer's disease, probably slightly less than Donepezil. Its mechanism of action is uncertain. It is not available on prescription and should only be taken with prescription drugs after taking medical advice.

Antidepressants

Antidepressants mostly act by restoring depleted levels of neurotransmitters. Many of the early antidepressants share a common biochemical structure of three rings and are referred to as 'tricyclics'. These include Amitriptyline, Imipramine, Dothiepin, Doxepin and Lofepramine. Their unwanted effects include drowsiness and sometimes a fall in blood pressure on standing up (postural hypotension), which can precipitate falls. Other unwanted tricyclic effects include dry mouth, confusion (caused by anti-cholinergic side-effects), constipation and occasionally the precipitation of eye disease (glaucoma) and retention of urine. Taken in overdose they can cause the heart to malfunction. Newer tricyclics like Lofepramine and other non-tricyclic antidepressants including the SSRIs have less of these side-effects, though they have their own problems. There is an increasing range of new antidepressants and here is not the place to discuss them in detail, but these include Venlafaxine. As many lack anti-cholinergic side-effects they are better suited to the treatment of depression and anxiety in people with dementia. They may be of particular benefit to people with depression in early dementia. Sometimes, in more advanced dementia, restlessness, agitation and other behavioural disturbance may be signs of an underlying depressed mood, which the patient is unable to report. Treatment with an SSRI or similar antidepressant may be reflected by reduced agitation and behaviour problems. When they are used in this way it is important to decide in advance what are the target symptoms or problems, so that after an appropriate period – between two and six weeks – an assessment can ascertain any benefit and a decision can be made about continuing treatment.

Another, older class of antidepressant is the monoamine oxidase inhibitors. Unfortunately, complicated dietary restrictions must be observed if they are to be taken safely, so they have little place in the treatment of the dementia sufferer. However, St John's Wort, a herbal remedy for depression with some demonstrated usefulness, is probably a mild monoamine oxidase inhibitor. It is not available on prescription in the UK and should not be used in combination with prescribed drugs without taking medical advice.

Antipsychotics

Antipsychotics – also called neuroleptics or 'major tranquillisers' – act mainly on the dopamine neurotransmitter systems in the brain. Their specific use is in schizophrenia. They include drugs like Chlorpromazine, Haloperidol, Thioridazine, Promazine and Trifluoperazine. They also have a non-specific use as sedatives and tranquillisers and it is for this that they are often used in restless patients with dementia. Because dopamine systems are also involved (in the extra-pyramidal nervous system) in Parkinson's disease, one of the common unwanted effects of antipsychotics is the induction of a Parkinsonian state characterised by stiffness, trembling, slowness of movement and sometimes, paradoxically, restlessness. A longer-term side-effect results in writhing movements of the tongue, face or body ('tardive dyskinesia'). Collectively the earlier and late-onset side-effects are known as extrapyramidal side-effects (EPSE). Some drugs, like Haloperidol and Trifluoperazine, produce particularly strong EPSE and so dosage has to be controlled very carefully. Others, such as Chlorpromazine and Thioridazine, are less likely to cause Parkinsonian effects, but may increase confusion and also may still cause tardive dyskinesia. Chlorpromazine in particular may also cause postural hypotension. Droperidol is related to Haloperidol and has a very marked sedative effect.

A new generation of 'atypical' antipsychotics is generally only licensed for the treatment of schizophrenia. This group includes Clozapine (which can only be used under special conditions), Risperidone, Olanzipine and Quetiapine. Because many have a low incidence of EPSE, psychiatrists sometimes use them to treat hallucinations and persecutory states associated with dementia. Conventional antipsychotics can be dangerous for patients with dementia with Lewy bodies, and if antipsychotics must be used most specialists will chose careful treatment with low-dose 'atypicals'.

Anxiolytics

Anxiolytics, also known as 'minor tranquillisers' and used as sleeping tablets, are commonly prescribed psychotropic drugs. Most of them belong to a group known as benzodiazepines and include Diazepam, Nitrazepam, Flurazepam, Temazepam, Lorazepam and Lormetazepam. Many old people use them to get to sleep, but they also have unwanted effects. They may accumulate and cause over-sedation or 'hangover' effects, and patients may become dependent on them. They may also impair memory and performance of complex motor tasks. They may be responsible for falls. There are now strong moves to restrict their prescribing to short-term use as the burden of disability caused by them is recognised. Other, newer forms of sleeping tablets should also only be used in the short term. Some of the newer SSRI antidepressants are licensed for use in various forms of anxiety disorders, and are generally better for this purpose than the benzodiazepines.

Drug metabolism and interactions

In old age there are changes in the way in which the body processes (metabolises) drugs that cannot be described in detail here. The effect of most of these changes is to render old people more susceptible to the unwanted effects of drugs and this, combined with multiple diseases and multiple prescriptions, puts old people at special risk of adverse drug effects. For a fuller description of metabolism and interactions and other medical and psychological aspects, see Wattis and Curran (in press).

Specific problems

Sleeplessness and night-time restlessness

It is important to exclude specific causes of sleeplessness, for example, pain, heart failure and depression. If these are present they should be treated. Catnaps during the day should be avoided. Adequate exercise and mental stimulation should be provided during the day, and stimulant drinks, including coffee and tea, kept to a minimum in the evening. A small warm milky drink and a clear bedtime routine may help. There should not be an unrealistically early bedtime or unrealistic expectations of how long the old person with dementia will sleep. Emotional and practical support to the carer may also reduce the emotional burden of disturbed nights. When all these measures have been tried, there will remain a minority of demented old people whose night-time restlessness is intolerable to the caregiver. In these circumstances, low doses of the more sedative major tranquillisers, such as 10 to 25 mg Thioridazine in the late evening, may be useful. If there is evidence of possible depressed mood, then a sedative antidepressant such as Trazodone may be given at night and its effects carefully monitored. Sometimes a benzodiazepine or other sleeping tablet may be useful for a limited period, usually for a maximum of a week.

Daytime restlessness and wandering

If there is a marked increase in daytime wandering or restlessness, causes must again be sought. Is the wandering secondary to depressed mood and consequent agitation? If there is depressed mood, this can be treated with an appropriate sedative antidepressant, such as Dothiepin or Trazodone. Often this can be given as a single night-time dose, when it has the bonus action of improving sleep. Once again, when all commonsense remedies have failed, the non-specific use of medication may be considered. Very low doses of Haloperidol – eg, 0.5 to 1 mg twice daily – or higher doses of Thioridazine – eg, 10 to 25 mg up to three times a day – may help, but should not generally be continued long term. In some cases low doses of atypical antipsychotics such as Risperidone 0.5 mg twice daily may be more appropriate. Minor tranquillisers are generally not much use in this situation.

Incontinence

Incontinence is rare until dementia is very advanced (except in unusual forms of dementia such as normal pressure hydrocephalus, or where there is a local cause such as a urine infection). In the earlier stages of dementia, toileting difficulties are frequently due to such problems as failure to find the toilet, or to medical problems such as constipation or urinary tract infection, which must be tackled in their own right (see Chapter 11). Most drugs given to promote continence are likely to increase confusion and rarely contribute much to improving the incontinence.

Aggression and violence

Violence is rarely unpredictable. Martin Luther King once said (in quite a different context) that violence is the voice of the unheard. This aphorism also applies to the dementia sufferer. An old lady who believes she has to go home to make her (dead) husband's tea or attend to the baby is unlikely to take kindly to the staff member who blocks her way and tells her not to be so silly! This kind of behaviour is fortunately now much rarer among professionals of all disciplines, who are trained to try to understand the world from the demented patient's point of view and use a pleasant approach and techniques such as distraction and validation rather than authoritarian confrontation. With the best care in the world, some old people with dementia will occasionally become violent. Again it is important to consider whether there may be a medical cause – such as an infection or heart failure leading to a sudden increase in confusion (acute confusional state). Medication may be needed in an emergency to contain the situation while other measures are taken. Low doses of Droperidol by mouth or, very rarely if ever, intramuscular Haloperidol may be justified. Such measures should always be regarded as short-term until better approaches can be devised. In short-staffed long-stay facilities, there may be a temptation to use sedative medication to make life more manageable for the staff. This is a difficult ethical problem for the doctor who often feels powerless to influence staffing levels, but does not believe in using sedation to compensate for lack of staff time. The only real solution is the provision of adequate numbers of well trained staff.

Conclusion

The medical management of dementia demands an accurate diagnosis. There are now some specific treatments for Alzheimer's disease as well as measures that may reduce the risk of multi-infarct dementia developing or progressing. When it comes to symptomatic treatment of problem behaviours, it is essential to try to determine and deal with underlying causes. Often such behaviours are the result of an inappropriate environment, over-stressed carers, physical illness or discomfort and are best dealt with by addressing the underlying problems. Depression may co-exist with dementia, and the newer antidepressants give better opportunities for treating depression and associated behaviour disturbance in dementia. Sedative medication is only one of a range of alternative approaches and, because of the possibility of unwanted effects, should be reserved until other measures have been tried and found to be ineffective.

References
Wattis J & Curran S, (in press), *Practical Psychiatry of Old Age* (3rd edn), Radcliffe Press, Oxford.

CHAPTER 20

Supporting the Families of People with Dementia

Marie Claire Shankland

THE CARE OF MOST PEOPLE WITH DEMENTIA takes place in the community, as approximately four out of five people with dementia are living outside hospital or residential settings. Although some of these individuals live alone (mainly those in their late eighties and nineties), the majority live with a member of their family – usually their spouse, but sometimes their son or daughter. Since the average time from the onset of Alzheimer's disease until death is between five and 10 years, with about four of these spent at home, a considerable burden of caring is shouldered by family members. The Carers (Recognition and Services) Act (Department of Health, 1995) lays out the rights of carers to have their role recognised and to have their needs assessed and met.

The challenges of caring

Unlike other terminal illnesses, people suffering from dementia not only undergo physical changes, but also changes in personality and intellect. Family carers have to cope with both practical tasks and the loss of their loved one, as they have known them.

Often just knowing what the illness is can ease the strain on families. Before diagnosis is made and information about the illness is given, people will often blame the person with dementia or assume their difficult behaviour is deliberate and under their control. It is important to take care to find out if the diagnosis has been shared and information given about the illness, what to expect and how to understand difficult behaviour. However, even once the diagnosis has been established, the challenges of supporting someone with dementia are varied and burdensome.

A substantial amount of research has been done which illustrates the particular strain of caring for someone with dementia (Zarit & Edwards, 1996). It is vital to realise that carer stress is not a simple matter: it is a mixture of complex circumstances, relationships, responses and different coping styles, which often change over the course of the illness (Pearlin *et al*, 1990).

Problems experienced by carers

The most frequent problems reported by those caring for people with dementia include:

- Inability of the dependant to be left alone
- Disruption of the carer's personal life
- Inability to hold a conversation with the person
- Lack of self-help skills, such as dressing, feeding and bathing
- Loss of sexual intimacy and emotional support from the person
- Repetitive questioning
- Incontinence
- Demands for attention.

Changes in family relationships

The nature of the previous relationship seems crucial in understanding how the carer will cope with dementia in a loved one. Some of the reactions to caregiver burden can be seen as grief reactions to the gradual and fluctuating loss of their loved one. If a couple have been extremely close, that person is losing their companion, confidante, lover and friend. They can experience feelings of loneliness and being lost, which in some cases can lead to feelings of depression (Morris *et al*, 1988). However, if relationships in the family have been strained or abusive, people can experience feelings of conflict, guilt and resentment about having to care for the person.

People caring for someone with dementia will often tell us that friends and family find the illness very difficult to come to terms with, and thus carers may find themselves increasingly socially isolated. Sometimes this is because the main carer tries to protect the dignity of the person with dementia and no longer takes them into situations in which they would behave inappropriately, or be overwhelmed. Friends and family are often embarrassed and frightened and choose not to visit or invite the person with dementia and the carer any more. It is important when supporting families to find out what the support network is like, and we should work to maximise the support from the social network. Sometimes this means meeting with friends and family to explain more about the illness, or helping the main carer to discuss and negotiate with family and friends to gain their support. Flexible services for the person with dementia should take into account social and family networks and work alongside them.

Combating isolation and stimulating social support are key to carers maintaining morale and continuing in the caring role. Sadly, for both the person with dementia and their carer, being able to maintain friendship is limited when forgetfulness and communication problems develop. Allowing people to grieve for the changes in their loved one is crucial to supporting family carers.

Coping with caring at home

Carers have different ways of coping with caring. For some it seems that gathering information, making use of services such as day care, home help, mobile meals and drawing on family support help most. For others, 'psychological' strategies are important. These include finding an explanation for the illness and emphasising the positive side of the situation. Indeed, workers often underestimate the importance of the rewarding aspects of caregiving. Carers will often say that trying to cope with the illness together brings a couple closer, and sons and daughters will often comment that this is an opportunity to repay parents for the care they received as children.

Satisfaction with caring has been identified as important in enabling carers to continue their role (Nolan *et al*, 1996). Helping people to maintain positive elements of their relationship, for example by focusing on how they can continue to communicate and share things together, is as important as dealing with practical problems, respite and financial issues.

Denial that there is an illness is a strategy used by some carers; problems such as forgetfulness are attributed to 'old age', and sometimes specialist services will be refused. This is more likely to happen if carers have been struggling to cope for a while without support, or if the support offered does not meet the needs they have identified for themselves. On a more negative front, ignoring the relative with dementia and withdrawing from caring can also occur. Trying to force the carer back into this role is unlikely to be effective. It is important that those working with families recognise that there will be differences in people's coping strategies and in how they view their capacity to care. The approach is not to dictate how people should cope, but to maximise their range of coping strategies or help plan alternative care. For instance, information and one-to-one pre-diagnostic counselling may be more suitable than a relatives' support group to a carer who has not acknowledged the illness. Home-based respite from a community support worker may be better than residential respite care for a carer who wants one afternoon off a week.

The key to getting it right for carers is to make a thorough assessment of the things they are finding easy to cope with and the things that they find challenging and distressing. We know that men and women cope in different ways, and that services often provide men with more practical support while assuming that women can cope with practicalities. Such assumptions are unhelpful and often cause carers to withdraw from our offers of help. It is helpful to assess whether carers need practical support, some time away from their relative, or someone to talk to about their distress. Often support that we would see as minimal, such as the opportunity to go out once a week to visit friends for an hour, can be crucial to a carer and more worthwhile than regular day care which upsets the person with dementia and leads to struggles and arguments.

Physical dependence
Physical dependence is better tolerated by families than the challenge and strain of disruptive behaviour. This may be due to the fact that task-centred activities are easier for the carer to cope with emotionally. Repetitive questioning and uncooperative behaviour can be a constant

worry and strain, and it can be difficult to learn how to approach such behaviour. However, some partners and families find the intimacy of physical care shocking and will need practical support from services.

Abuse

The strain on carers, both emotional and physical, can put both carer and dependant at risk. Physical and emotional abuse of older people by carers is an under-researched area. One survey estimated that 500,000 elderly people are at risk of abuse from carers. Sexual abuse is not unknown. In some cases spouses will feel aware that they may be exploiting and taking advantage of a partner who is unable to say 'no'. Equally, carers find it very difficult to ask for help when a partner has become sexually aggressive or has raped them. Professionals need to be sensitive to the possibilities of abuse occurring and may have to raise difficult issues with carers.

Helping carers

How then can professionals working with people with dementia and their families help to meet their needs? Flexibility of approach is vital. Traditional models of carer support have viewed them as co-clients, co-workers or superceded carers (to be encouraged to take respite and ultimately give up the caring role to professional carers in a residential setting). An alternative model is to view the carer *and* the client as the experts. They have already been adjusting, thinking and coping long before services have become involved. It is also important to acknowledge that the dementing process and the involvement of caring professionals invades the privacy of people's closest relationship and rightly carers often react against such an invasion. People often feel very guilty about not being able to cope and shy away from asking for help. It is vital to reassure people that many of the feelings and failures they experience are because this illness is extremely difficult to cope with and not a reflection on their best efforts. A thorough assessment of people's circumstances is vital to being able to offer support that a carer is likely to find helpful. Carers will reject support that is not helpful and may become alienated from services only re-presenting in a crisis. Most carers state that it is helpful, if no help is required initially, to a have a point of contact for the future, so they need not re-tell their story repeatedly to different professionals before getting help.

Case Study 20.1 illustrates how supporting the carer as an expert can establish a relationship that helps the family to keep their loved one at home.

Case Study 20.1 Supporting Mrs Jones

Mrs Jones had been caring for her husband who had been diagnosed one year previously with probable Alzheimer's disease. Her husband was becoming increasingly distressed, following her around the house, asking to go home and asking who she was. Mrs Jones was unable to get any peace in the house while he was awake. Her daughter and family had visited for half-term week and she was horrified by the situation. This had led to the daughter arguing with her brother who lived close by their mother, and the daughter going to the general practitioner (GP) to demand something was done. Mrs Jones was extremely upset about all this and reluctant to allow anyone to visit for fear her husband would be put in a home. On visiting it was important at the outset to acknowledge that it must have been upsetting to have the visit forced upon her by the family. Mrs Jones was then able to explain that she had been trying very hard to keep her husband's condition from her children because they adored him and would be devastated by it. She had known for many months that she was struggling, but felt inadequate and knew her husband would have wanted the problem kept in the family. Mrs Jones had seen their elderly neighbour taken into care when she was confused and felt the lady had just given up and died – she did not want this to happen to her husband. Together it was agreed that a befriender would be introduced to the couple with a view to her going out one morning a week to visit her sister, and for her to have one morning alone in the house. It was also agreed that she needed to talk to her children to let them know more about their father's illness and to negotiate some help from them at weekends, and possibly to organise a family holiday. Mrs Jones was, in fact, handling her husband's difficult behaviour very well, and in addition to reinforcing her good work it was suggested that perhaps her husband felt afraid a lot of the time. Mrs Jones was also then able to comfort her husband, and in time this reduced his following and questioning behaviour.

Families and residential care

Families often experience tremendous guilt over the issue of admitting a loved one into residential or hospital care, and may feel embarrassed and harshly judged by others, as revealed by comments such as: 'I felt that I had let her down. We'd always been so close. But I've had two heart attacks and some days I can barely get myself, let alone my wife, out of bed.' 'My dad did so much for me, but they said it was clear I couldn't cope with him and I had to let him go in. I'm so ashamed I let him down.'

The cause of infrequent visiting may be that relatives experience grief and guilt on these occasions and feel unable to disclose this. Professionals need to be aware of this and provide time for relatives to voice such feelings, particularly when arrangements for residential care are being made. Staff in hospital and residential homes can encourage relatives to continue to be involved at a level they feel comfortable with. Even today many carers report they felt unwelcome and 'in the way', and in some cases have even been discouraged from visiting by staff. They can feel they have been 'superceded' as carers by nurses and support workers. Even if they wish to, few carers ask to take their relatives home for the day or for short visits because they fear interfering with the work of the home. Having the person with dementia home for a birthday or family celebration can mean a lot to carers.

Thus it is not only important to provide carers with emotional support while they are caring for their relative; it is also vital to help them with the transition between home and permanent care, and to maintain the link with them as 'family carers' following admission. Some carers, however, do wish the admission into care to be the end of their involvement and this must also be respected.

Meeting the needs of carers

Services available to help people with dementia and their carers vary from place to place. What suits one family may not be helpful for another. However, the following have been found to be of help by different individuals.

Carer support groups

These have become a popular way of offering some support and advice to carers of people with dementia. There are three main kinds of support group: those designed to provide practical information for carers about services, medication, moving and handling, looking after financial affairs and problem-solving; those that focus on stress management techniques for the carer, such as relaxation, problem-solving, anger control and anxiety management, and those that focus on teaching carers techniques to change the behaviour of the person with dementia in order to give the carer a greater sense of control and, hopefully, to increase their self-confidence. The evidence would suggest that carers appreciate attending groups, and find it useful to meet other people in the same situation, which helps them to feel less lonely and isolated. However, groups vary in their success in addressing symptoms of stress, anxiety and depression in carers. Before setting up groups it is important to decide their purpose, and to consider what the target of the group is – whether it is a social, informational or amore therapeutic, emotion-focused group.

For any carer group to be successful, carers need to be able to attend regularly. This will involve providing transport and respite services such as sitters to ensure the carer feels their relative is taken care of. Spouse carers will often prefer morning groups in order to be home in time for their spouse coming home from day care. Those caring for a parent or a younger person with dementia may wish to have evening groups due to work commitments. It is also important to provide refreshments for carers and to make them feel welcomed and looked after. Carers will often comment that coming to the group is the only time anyone does something for them.

Whether the group is educational in its focus or not it is important to have lots of local information on services, benefits and local carer organisations like the Alzheimer's Society, because carers often find this information difficult to find.

Comfort is also important and it is good to remember that many older people will have hearing and visual impairments and may have problems that make sitting still for long periods painful. Carers will often drop out of groups for very practical reasons like not being able to get up the stairs or being unable to hear what others say. It is also important to start and finish promptly, as carers' free time is precious.

If the support group is to be time-limited it is helpful to consider what support carers will have after the group finishes. With permanent support groups it is important to review how they are going from time to time as such groups often become purposeless. Either way it is important to ask the carers regularly how they find the group and how it can be improved.

Finally, it is useful to remember that groups may be particularly needed after the person with dementia has been admitted to care. It is essential that such a group addresses the feelings of grief and guilt carers experience at that time.

Respite care

Attendance at day centres for people with dementia and regular one- or two-week stays in hospital, local authority or private nursing homes are often suggested to, or requested by, carers. However, the needs of the person with dementia need to be taken into account too. What will be the effect of time spent away from home? In some cases disorientation and confusion may be increased after a residential stay, with a consequent increase in demands on the carer. Where day care is concerned, although a break for the carer may be crucial, the kind of stimulation offered to the person with dementia must be considered. Some day care provision merely provides a meal and a safe environment, but offers no therapeutic activity that may be of positive benefit. Often the levels of staff needed to care and provide therapeutic activity for people with dementia are too low.

Weekend and night respite (particularly for those caring for sufferers who are alert and wakeful at night) may be of more value to some carers than weekday day care. Likewise the opportunity to use a respite bed for a person with dementia one week per month or every six weeks may be preferable to permanent care. It is important to consult with local carers when planning services, in order that they meet their needs, and not to assume that service providers know what they require.

Domiciliary support

As has already been mentioned, the needs of the person with dementia have to be considered alongside those of the carers. Some people with dementia have been lifelong loners or simply prefer to stay at home. Care in the home is often quoted by the carer and person with dementia as their preferred option. Many carers reject the offer of home care or sitting services because they claim that they do not need help with housework.

Home care services work best when they are focused on helping the person with dementia with activities of daily living and simple domestic routines, in order that the carer can have a break in or out of the home. The key to this being successful is that the home care worker builds up a trusting relationship with the person with dementia. Sitting services can also be helpful where someone will sit with the person with dementia if they cannot be left alone while the carer goes out to shop or meet socially. Sitting services are provided by both voluntary and statutory agencies.

Advice, counselling and therapy
Carers should have access via their GP to teams of professionals experienced in dealing with dementia care. Once in contact with services, carers should have a named individual and phone number that they can use when they need help and advice. Carer support and advice is also available through the Alzheimer's society. Individual or family therapy or counselling should also be available through specialist teams.

Conclusion
To summarise, it should be possible for a package of care to be arranged which makes use of available services and takes into account the needs of both the carer and the person with dementia. Flexible care arrangements, continued counselling and involvement with other carers should also be available for families who have a relative in permanent residential or hospital care. Professionals need to be aware of all the services available in a particular area, and to know who to contact to discuss providing them. Integration of services and flexibility are crucial to helping carers cope.

References
Department of Health, 1995, Carers (Recognition and Services) Act, Policy Guidance, London.

Morris LW, Morris RG & Britton PG, 1988, 'The relationship between marital intimacy, perceived strain and depression in spouse caregivers of dementia sufferers', *British Journal of Medical Psychology* 61, pp231–6.

Nolan M, Grant G & Keady J, 1996, *Understanding Family Care*, Open University Press, Buckingham.

Pearlin LI, Mullan JT, Semple SJ & Skaff MM, 1990, 'Caregiving and the stress process: an overview of concepts and their measures', *Gerontologist* 30(5), pp583–94.

Zarit SH and Edwards AB, 1996, 'Family Caregiving: Research and Clinical Intervention', Woods RT (ed), *Handbook of Clinical Psychology of Ageing*, Chichester: John Wiley.